T0074121

Imaging Tumor Response to Therapy

Massimo Aglietta • Daniele Regge

Editors

Imaging Tumor Response to Therapy

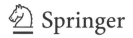

Editors
Massimo Aglietta
Department of Medical Oncology
University of Turin
Institute for Cancer Research
and Treatment (IRCC)
Candiolo (Turin)
Italy

Daniele Regge
Radiology Unit
Institute for Cancer Research
and Treatment (IRCC)
Candiolo (Turin)
Italy

ISBN 978-88-470-2612-4   e-ISBN 978-88-470-2613-1

DOI 10.1007/978-88-470-2613-1

Springer Milan Dordrecht Heidelberg London New York

Library of Congress Control Number: 2012939431

5 4 3 2 1   2012   2013   2014   2015

Cover design: Ikona S.r.l., Milan, Italy
Typesetting: Graphostudio, Milan, Italy
Printing and binding: Grafiche Porpora, Segrate (Milan), Italy

Printed in Italy

Springer-Verlag Italia S.r.l. – Via Decembrio 28 – I-20137 Milan
Springer is a part of Springer Science+Business Media (www.springer.com)

Measure what is measurable,
and make measurable what is not so.
Galileo Galilei

Preface

The first drugs for cancer chemotherapy became available more than 50 years ago. At that time, these chemotherapeutic agents were observed to produce tumor shrinkage and thus, in some cases, increased survival and even patient cure. The identification of a potentially active therapy followed a very simple scheme: a treatment producing a significant reduction of the tumor burden in a consistent percentage of patients (generally > 20%) was considered active and thus most likely able to improve survival. Later, the need to anticipate the response to treatment drove researchers to determine a measure that could be used as a surrogate for a clinically meaningful endpoint. Accordingly, in 1979–1981 the World Health Organization produced a set of imaging criteria to monitor the response to treatment of patients enrolled in clinical trials, based on measurement of the longest lesion diameter. In 2000, a set of new rules to define tumor response was published, the Response Evaluation Criteria in Solid Tumors (RECIST), by the European Organization for Research and Treatment of Cancer (EORTC) and the National Cancer Institute.

Today, in addition to the numerous chemotherapeutic agents, new targeted-therapy drugs are available, often used to treat the same disease as their predecessors. Their mechanism of action is complex such that the dogma *tumor shrinkage = activity* does not always hold true. Instead, targeted drugs are able to stabilize disease, which can increase patient survival and/or quality of life to a greater extent than agents inducing a transient tumor shrinkage. Moreover, particularly with some of the new agents that target specific molecular pathways, there is evidence that tumor growth is strongly inhibited even if there is no change or a paradoxical increase in tumor volume is observed at conventional imaging. Thus, in clinical practice the decision whether or not to consider a treatment effective may be challenging.

These problems are amplified during drug development, when critical decisions are made regarding the value of further efforts. Improved patient survival, the true endpoint, is inappropriate in early clinical trials and even in randomized phase III studies it is often difficult to determine because of the confounding effect of sequential treatments. Thus, surrogate endpoints of activity have become crucial.

The appreciation that a simple dimensional evaluation of the tumor might be inappropriate or misleading has also forced oncologists and radiologists to establish more effective and straightforward criteria to define the activity and effects of treatment. This problem is addressed in this volume and, although it is not solved, we hope that the detailed discussion of specific clinical situations can contribute and enhance the ongoing debate.

Massimo Aglietta and Daniele Regge

Contents

Contributors

Ileana Baldi Department of Environmental Medicine and Public Health, University of Padua, Padua, Italy

Massimo Bellomi Department of Radiology, European Institute of Oncology, Milan; Department of Medicine and Surgery, University of Milan, Milan, Italy

Ilaria Bertotto Radiology Unit, Institute for Cancer Research and Treatment (IRCC), Candiolo (Turin), Italy

Paola Boccone Division of Medical Oncology, Institute for Cancer Research and Treatment (IRCC), Candiolo (Turin), Italy

Franco Brunello Gastro-Hepatology, San Giovanni Battista Hospital, Turin, Italy

Delia Campanella Radiology Unit, Institute for Cancer Research and Treatment (IRCC), Candiolo (Turin), Italy

Lorenzo Capussotti Surgical Department, Division of Hepato-Bilio-Pancreatic and Digestive Surgery, Mauriziano "Umberto I" Hospital, Turin, Italy

Giovannino Ciccone Unit of Clinical Epidemiology, San Giovanni Battista University Hospital and CPO Piemonte, Turin, Italy

Stefano Cirillo Division of Radiology, Mauriziano "Umberto I" Hospital, Turin, Italy

Francesco De Cobelli Department of Radiology, San Raffaele Hospital and Experimental Imaging Center, Vita-Salute University, Milan, Italy

Tommaso De Pas Medical Oncology Unit of Respiratory Tract and Sarcomas New Drugs, Development Division, European Institute of Oncology, Milan, Italy

Alessandro Del Maschio Department of Radiology, San Raffaele Hospital and Experimental Imaging Center, Vita-Salute University, Milan, Italy

Angelo S. Del Sole Department of Biomedical Science and Technology, University of Milan, Nuclear Medicine, San Paolo Hospital, Milan, Italy

Nadia Di Muzio Department of Radiotherapy, San Raffaele Hospital, Milan, Italy

Anastassia Esseridou Department of Radiology, IRCCS Policlinico San Donato, San Donato Milanese (Mi), Italy

Giovanni Grignani Division of Medical Oncology, Institute for Cancer Research and Treatment (IRCC), Candiolo (Turin), Italy

Francesco Leone Department of Medical Oncology, University of Turin, Institute for Cancer Research and Treatment (IRCC), Candiolo (Turin), Italy

Claudio Losio Department of Radiology, San Raffaele Hospital, Milan, Italy

Laura Martincich Radiology Unit, Institute for Cancer Research and Treatment (IRCC), Candiolo (Turin), Italy

Filippo Montemurro Division of Medical Oncology, Institute for Cancer Research and Treatment (IRCC), Candiolo (Turin), Italy

Marcello Orsi Department of Radiology, San Raffaele Hospital, Milan, Italy

Cinzia Ortega Division of Medical Oncology, Institute for Cancer Research and Treatment (IRCC), Candiolo (Turin), Italy; Italian Nephro-Oncology Group (G.I.O.N.)

Camillo Porta Division of Medical Oncology, IRCCS San Matteo University Hospital Foundation, Pavia, Italy; Italian Nephro-Oncology Group (G.I.O.N.)

Lorenzo Preda Department of Radiology, European Institute of Oncology, Milan, Italy

Michele Reni Department of Oncology, San Raffaele Hospital, Milan, Italy

Manuela Racca Nuclear Medicine Unit, Institute for Cancer Research and Treatment (IRCC), Candiolo (Turin), Italy

Filippo Russo Radiology Unit, Institute for Cancer Research and Treatment (IRCC), Candiolo (Turin), Italy

Francesco Sardanelli Department of Medical Surgical Sciences, University of Milan, Department of Radiology, IRCCS Policlinico San Donato, San Donato Milanese (Mi), Italy

Luca M. Sconfienza Department of Radiology, IRCCS Policlinico San Donato, San Donato Milanese (Mi), Italy

Adele Tessitore Department of Thoracic Surgery, European Institute of Oncology, Milan, Italy

Teresio Varetto Nuclear Medicine Unit, Institute for Cancer Research and Treatment (IRCC), Candiolo (Turin), Italy

Andrea Veltri Department of Radiology, Facoltà San Luigi Gonzaga, University of Turin, Orbassano (Turin), Italy

Luca Viganò Surgical Department, Division of Hepato-Bilio-Pancreatic and Digestive Surgery, Mauriziano "Umberto I" Hospital, Turin, Italy

Abbreviations

^{18}F-FAZA	^{18}F-fluoroazomycin arabinoside
^{18}F-FDG	^{18}F-fluorodeoxyglucose
^{18}F-FLT	^{18}F-fluorothymidine
^{18}F-FMISO	^{18}F-fluoromisonidazole
^{18}F-RGD	^{18}F-galacto-arginine-glycine-aspartic acid
1D	one-dimensional
2D	two-dimensional
3D	three-dimensional
4D	four-dimensional
AASLD	American Association for the Study of Liver Diseases
ADC	apparent diffusion coefficient
AUC	area under the curve
BCLC	Barcelona Clinic of Liver Cancer
CA	carbohydrate antigen
CAST	cardiac arrhythmia suppressing trial
CDDP	chemotherapy containing cisplatin
CEA	carcinoembryonic antigen
CEUS	contrast-enhanced ultrasound
CR	complete response
CRC	colorectal cancer
CT	computed tomography
DCE	dynamic contrast-enhanced
DCE-MRI	dynamic contrast-enhanced MRI
DCE-US	dynamic contrast-enhanced ultrasound
DFS	disease-free survival
DWI	diffusion-weighted imaging
DW-MRI	diffusion-weighted magnetic resonance imaging
EASL	European Association for the Study of the Liver
EES	extracellular extravascular space
EFS	event-free survival
EGFR	epidermal growth factor receptor

EORTC	European Organization for Research and Treatment of Cancer
ESPAC	European Study Group for Pancreatic Cancer
FA	folinic acid
FDA	Food and Drug Administration
FU	5-fluorouracil
GCB	gemcitabine
GIST	gastrointestinal stromal tumor
GITSG	Gastro Intestinal Tumor Study Group
GLUT	glucose transporters
HCC	hepatocellular carcinoma
HIF	hypoxia inducible factor
HR	hazard ratio
HU	Hounsfield unit
IAUGC	initial area under the gadolinium concentration
IFN-α	interferon-α
IPD	individual patient data
IRA	iodine-related attenuation
LBM	lean body mass
LUF	lipoidol ultrafluid
LV	leucovorin
MAPK	mitogen-activated protein kinase
MASS	mass, attenuation, size and structure
mCRC	metastatic CRC
MDCT	multi-detector CT
mRECIST	modified RECIST assessment
MRI	magnetic resonance imaging
MRS	magnetic resonance spectroscopy
mTOR	mammalian target of rapamycin
MX	mammography
NAC	neoadjuvant chemotherapy
NAT	neoadjuvant therapy
NSCLC	non-small-cell lung cancer
ORR	objective response rate
OS	overall survival
pCR	pathological complete response
PCT	primary chemotherapy
PD	progressive disease
PDGF	platelet-derived growth factor
PDGFR	PDGF receptors
PET	positron emission tomography
PFS	progression-free survival
PR	partial response
PSA	prostate-specific antigen
RCC	renal cell carcinoma
RCTs	randomized controlled trials

RECICL	Response Evaluation Criteria in Cancer of the Liver
RECIST	Response Evaluation Criteria in Solid Tumors
ROI	region of interest
SACT	size and attenuation CT
SD	stable disease
SIR	Society of Interventional Radiology
STE	surrogate threshold effect
SUV	standardized uptake value
T/N ratio	tumor-to-normal tissue ratio
TACE	transhepatic arterial chemoembolization
TAE	transarterial embolization
TARE	transarterial 90Y radioembolization
TKI	tyrosine kinase inhibitor
TRK	tyrosine kinase
TTP	time to progression
TTT	time to next treatment
US	ultrasound
VEGF	vascular endothelial growth factor
VEGFRs	VEGF receptors
VHL	von Hippel-Lindau
WHO	World Health Organization

Part I
Methodological Bases

Surrogate Endpoints of Clinical Benefit

1

Giovannino Ciccone and Ileana Baldi

1.1   Introduction

Despite several decades of intensive clinical and biological research and significant progress in primary prevention, screening, diagnosis, prognosis, and treatment, cancer is still the second most common cause of death in developed countries, accounting for about one-fourth of total deaths [1]. Accordingly, an improvement in the prognosis of cancer patients is a powerful stimulus for researchers, regulatory agencies, and the health care industry and, of course, a high priority for patients and society. Similar to the HIV/AIDS community, there have been numerous efforts to accelerate approvals of new drugs but also to shorten the times required in their development and marketing, with positive as well as negative consequences.

It is widely accepted that the ultimate goal of any health care intervention should be an average net benefit for those treated, with a favorable balance between desirable and unwanted consequences. However, while there are few difficulties in measuring the risks (at least the most frequent ones and those with a short latency) and the costs of a particular treatment, defining and measuring the benefits can be problematic. Since most cancer treatments, especially chemotherapies, have safety risks, a necessary condition that must be satisfied for a patient to accept treatment is that improvement in terms of relevant and reliable clinical benefits will outweigh the harm done by the treatment. In addition, from a societal perspective, the acceptability and the economic and organizational sustainability of treatment have gained in importance. Direct measures of how a patient feels, is able to function, or whether he or she survives following treatment are considered the only definite and

G. Ciccone (✉)
Unit of Clinical Epidemiology, San Giovanni Battista University Hospital and CPO Piemonte,
Turin, Italy

M. Aglietta, D. Regge (eds.), *Imaging Tumor Response to Therapy,* © Springer-Verlag Italia 2012

meaningful endpoints of clinical benefit. Therefore, it would be logical to expect that most of the evidence provided by clinical research would be based on measures of definite clinical benefit important to the patients, expressed in terms of gains in survival and in the quality of life. However, the majority of the new drugs registered for cancer treatment in the last several years rely on *surrogate endpoints*, i.e., indirect measures of definite or true clinical benefits. The widespread use of surrogate endpoints in clinical research, in regulatory processes, and in practice is often justified and addresses many interests, but it is also accompanied by frequent misconceptions as well as legitimate concerns about the potential harm deriving from the application of preliminary results based on surrogates and without adequate validation. The recent report of the Institute of Medicine "Evaluation of Biomarkers and Surrogate Endpoints in Chronic Disease," along with a thorough review of the literature, has provided robust recommendations for biomarker evaluation, implementation of the evaluation framework, supporting evidence-based decision making, and promoting public health [2].

In this chapter, we present some of the most widely used definitions of surrogate endpoints, with a discussion of the advantages as well as the risks connected with their use in research, in regulatory decisions, and in practice. We then address, with a more formal approach, the issue of their validation from a methodological perspective, which represents the heart of the problem. Finally, we derive from the literature and our own clinical experience a few recommendations to promote greater awareness regarding the use of surrogate endpoints within a clinical trial and in practice.

1.2 Definitions of Surrogate Endpoints

Surrogate endpoints, also called intermediate endpoints, surrogate markers, or biomarkers, comprise laboratory, imaging, and physical measurements considered as suitable substitutes for a clinically meaningful endpoint. There are several definitions of a surrogate endpoint in the literature, most of which have a statistical or regulatory origin.

The most often-quoted definition of a surrogate endpoint was proposed by Prentice [3], in a landmark paper on statistical evaluation methods. A surrogate endpoint was defined as "a response variable for which a test of the null hypothesis of no relationship to the treatment groups under comparison is also a valid test of the corresponding null hypothesis based on the true outcome." A frequently cited definition is that of Temple [4], who defined a surrogate endpoint of a clinical trial as "… a laboratory measurement or a physical sign used as a substitute for a clinically meaningful endpoint that measures directly how a patient feels, functions or survives. Changes introduced by a therapy on a surrogate endpoint are expected to reflect changes in a clinically meaningful endpoint." Another definition, proposed by the Biomarker Definitions Working Group [5], is: "a biomarker that is intended to substitute for a clinical endpoint. A surrogate endpoint is expected to predict clinical benefit (or harm or lack of benefit or harm) based on epidemiologic, therapeutic, patho-physiologic, or other scientific evidence."

The common meaning of the available definitions is that "the treatment effect observed on a valid surrogate endpoint (substitute) should reliably and precisely predict the treatment effect on the clinical endpoint (entity being replaced)" [6], but the underlying necessary condition is that the surrogate endpoint must be validated with a rigorous methodology to prevent potential harm due to its imprudent use.

1.3   Potentials and Limits of Surrogate Endpoints

There are several reasons behind the widespread use of surrogate endpoints as primary measures of efficacy in research, in place of the true measure of clinical benefit. In oncology, overall survival (OS) is considered the gold standard, i.e., the highest endpoint in a hierarchy of importance, but its use as a primary endpoint is almost never considered for early-phase studies and only in a small proportion of randomized (phase III) controlled trials (RCTs). In most trials, to detect a clinically meaningful and statistically significant difference in OS, the required sample sizes, length of follow-up, and associated costs are often considered to be unaffordable. In addition, especially in diseases with a fair or good prognosis, OS may be influenced by the sequence of different treatments, thereby hampering estimates of the contribution of the experimental therapy, which usually affects only one step in the treatment pathway. The choice of an alternative, surrogate, endpoint, i.e., one that considers events more frequent than death, is more sensitive to the study treatment, and requires a shorter follow-up, is an obvious solution to obtain valuable results quickly and with fewer costs. However, this reasoning holds only if the surrogate endpoint is a valid substitute for the true endpoint of clinical benefit, thereby shifting attention to the causal pathway between treatment, surrogate and true endpoints, and thus to the validation problem.

The basic model of the causal pathway linking treatment to the true clinical endpoint assumes that the surrogate is an intermediate in the only causal pathway of the disease process, i.e., the intervention's entire effect on the true clinical outcome is mediated through its effect on the surrogate. However, there are several possible alternatives to this basic model. Thus, Fleming and DeMets [7] hypothesized that: (a) a surrogate endpoint, even if it correlates with clinical outcome, might not involve the same pathophysiological process contributing to that outcome; (b) among the disease pathways affecting the true clinical outcome, the intervention may only affect the pathway mediated through the surrogate endpoint, but not other mechanisms; (c) alternatively, treatment might affect only a disease pathway independent of the surrogate endpoint; (d) and, most importantly, the intervention might also affect the true clinical outcome by unintended mechanisms of action that are independent of the disease process. These few scenarios are sufficient to point out an important consequence: given the high variability, and the limited knowledge, of the underlying biological mechanisms linking the treatment with the true clinical outcome, especially in an era of emerging targeted therapies, the role of a surrogate endpoint should be assessed and validated specifically for each disease and each class of drugs.

The validation of surrogate endpoints has received increasing attention due to the harm caused by treatments whose efficacy was assessed using non-validated surrogate endpoints. A review citing several examples of the failure of potential surrogate endpoints, with an estimate of the harm done to patients, was published by Grimes and Schultz [8]. Among the many reported examples, one of the best known is the Cardiac Arrhythmia Suppressing Trial (CAST). The clinical and biological rationale supporting the drugs investigated in that study was so convincing that many experts raised ethical concerns about the trial: since the occurrence of ventricular arrhythmias, a complication of an acute myocardial infarction, is associated with a fourfold increase in sudden death, the early administration of anti-arrhythmic drugs in patients who suffered an acute myocardial infarction should have a beneficial effect. The agents compared to placebo in that trial (encainide, flecainide and moricizine), already approved by the FDA for severe arrhythmias and used in clinical practice, showed a strong effect on the surrogate endpoint (the occurrence of ventricular arrhythmias) but this beneficial effect was outweighed by a large increase in sudden deaths, the true primary clinical endpoint. It has been estimated that in the USA more than 200,000 patients received these drugs, and thousands died needlessly [8].

There are several other examples of treatments whose efficacy was determined based on non-validated surrogate endpoints, thus leading to harmful consequences, such as (the surrogate endpoint are noted in parentheses): some lipid-lowering agents (laboratory markers), some anti-hypertensive drugs (arterial blood pressure), certain anti-glycemic interventions (glycemia, glycated hemoglobin), bone mineralizing drugs (bone densitometry), and some erythropoiesis-stimulating agents (anemia).

Surrogate endpoints, all disease-centered, are quite frequently used in cancer clinical trials. Tumor response, usually measured with imaging or laboratory techniques and classified according to explicit criteria, is the primary endpoint in most phase II trials, in which the main interest is to screen promising new treatments according to their activity and safety profile, before investing in large comparative trials. In RCTs, the most widely used primary endpoints are composite measures of death (all-cause or disease-specific) and other disease-specific events. They are expressed as time to event, from a pre-specified starting time (usually randomization) until disease recurrence (disease-free survival, DFS, typically used in an adjuvant setting), disease progression (progression-free survival, PFS), or the occurrence of the first of several predefined events (event-free survival, EFS). Other measures, mainly used as secondary endpoints, are estimates of velocity of response (time to response,

TTR), duration of response (time to progression, TTP), or the time required for further treatments (time to next treatment, TTT). This list could be easily extended and better defined according to the type of cancer and the clinical setting, but the most important issue common to all these endpoints is the necessity of a robust validation before their use in clinical practice.

In oncology, there are several examples of treatments with demonstrated efficacy only on the surrogate endpoints, with minimal, if any, beneficial effects on survival or with an uncertain balance between benefits and risks. Moreover, only a few of the surrogate endpoints currently used as primary outcomes in RCTs have been fully validated. A further problem shared by most of these surrogates is the risk of measurement errors, often leading to biased estimates of efficacy (especially in non-blinded trials without independent central reviews).

There is a growing literature on the results of validation studies of the surrogate endpoints commonly used as primary outcome measures in cancer trials. In the review of Shi and Sargent [6], limited to the most rigorous validations available for colorectal, breast, and prostate cancer surrogate endpoints, the response rate has never been demonstrated to be a reliable surrogate for survival in advanced disease. In colorectal cancer studies, PFS was shown to be a strong surrogate for survival, as was DFS in adjuvant studies. By contrast, PFS was not confirmed as a valid surrogate for advanced breast cancer. In prostate cancer trials, various measures of prostate-specific antigen (PSA), such as the PSA response or longitudinal PSA measurements, showed a strong prognostic value, but none of them were confirmed as valid surrogates for survival. These results underline the problem of relying on prognostic markers instead of valid surrogates in effectiveness trials.

The importance of evidence based on surrogates in regulatory processes clearly emerges in the Accelerated Approval regulation of the US Food and Drug Administration (FDA). A recent report [9] summarizes the available data covering all the indications of oncology products that had received an accelerated approval between December 1992 and July 2010. Unlike the regular approval process, which requires substantial evidence of clinical benefit (in terms of prolongation or improvement of life), accelerated approval accepts results in terms of a surrogate endpoint, even from single-arm trials, but requires that the manufacturer later conduct post-approval clinical trials to confirm the clinical benefit. The aim of the Accelerated Approval regulation is to make new drugs more rapidly available to patients with serious or life-threatening illnesses. The results of the FDA's accelerated approval for oncology drugs are summarized in Table 1.1. Over a period of about 18 years, 35 oncology drugs with 47 indications received an accelerated approval by the FDA. In about 75% (35/47) of the approved indications, the study endpoint was response rate; this figure was 96% (27/28) in single-arm studies and 42% in randomized trials. In the same period, 26 (55%) of the 47 accelerated approvals received a subsequent regular approval, 3 (6%) were rejected due to an inability to demonstrate clinical benefit, 4 (8.5%) are currently under FDA

Table 1.1 Results of the US FDA Accelerated Approval Process for 35 oncology drugs, by study design and endpoint used (1992–2010) (from [9])

	Study design		Total	
	Single arm trial	Randomized trial	N.	Percent
Number of indications approved	28	19	47	100.0
Endpoint for accelerated approval:				
• Response rate	27	8	35	74.5
• Progression-free survival	-	5[a]	5	10.6
• Disease-free survival	-	4[b]	4	8.5
• Time to progression	-	1	1	2.1
• Reduced toxicity	1	1	2	4.3
Regular approval status:				
• Converted to regular approval	15	11	26	55.3
• Failed regular approval	3	-	3	6.4
• Under FDA review	2	2	4	8.5
• Study not completed	8	6	14	29.8

[a]Includes one study that used time to progression as the endpoint.
[b]Includes one study that used the incidence rate as the endpoint.

review, and in 14 (30%) a confirmatory study was not completed. The primary endpoints used in the 26 confirmatory studies carried out to receive a regular approval were: OS (10/26, 38.5%), PFS or TTP (7/26, 27%), DFS (3/26, 11.5%), response rate (5/26, 19%), and cardiac safety (1/26, 4%). The median time interval between accelerated and regular approval for the 26 confirmed indications was 3.9 years (range: 0.8–12.6), with an average interval of 4.7 years. However, the proportion of indications with accelerated approval for which definitive confirmation is nonetheless lacking is 30% and in only 10 cases was regular approval based on studies confirming a better OS. It is noteworthy that in some cases the results of the surrogate endpoints used to obtain an accelerated approval were subsequently confirmed by other surrogates; this is indeed a slippery slope.

The above-described experience highlights the critical dilemma surrounding the role of surrogate endpoints in clinical research: on the one hand, they have the potential to make new therapies more rapidly available to patients, but on the other they carry the risk of disseminating useless or harmful treatments, with negative consequences for patients and contributing to the waste of scarce resources. Table 1.2 summarizes the major advantages and limitations of using surrogate endpoints.

Table 1.2 Major advantages and limitations of using surrogate endpoint in research, regulation, and practice

Advantages of surrogate endpoints
• Improved research efficiency, by reducing trial sample size, duration, and costs
• Rapid elimination of non-promising treatments (especially in early-phase trials)
• The demonstration of larger effect sizes and more statistically sound results
• The distinction of confounding from other lines of treatments
• Better patient accessibility to new, potentially effective treatments by quicker approvals (especially for serious illness, when effective treatments are lacking)
Limitations or risks of surrogate endpoints
• In regulatory processes, to substitute true clinical endpoints with surrogates lacking sufficient validation
• Favors the diffusion of treatments with an overly optimistic balance between benefits (measured only with surrogates) and risks (with an underestimation of late toxicity)
• Potentially limited possibility of reliable cost-effectiveness evaluations
• Prevents or discourages investments in large, pragmatic, clinical trials with true clinical endpoints
• Higher risks of biased measurements (especially by observer assessments in non-blinded studies)
• The tendency to easily generalize the use of validated surrogates in different contexts (such as disease stage or severity, other drug classes)

1.4   Statistical Methods for the Validation of Surrogate Endpoints

Surrogate endpoints have an increasingly important role in clinical research, regulatory processes, and practice; however, their validation poses many statistical challenges.

From a statistical standpoint, according to the definitions proposed by Buyse [10], a *validated marker* is one that has been demonstrated by robust statistical methods to forecast the likely response to a treatment (predictive biomarker) or to be able to replace a clinical endpoint in assessing the effect of a treatment (surrogate endpoint). Despite the potential of surrogate endpoints, there is no widely accepted agreement about what constitutes a valid surrogate endpoint. In early discussions on this subject, a common misconception was that it was sufficient for the endpoint to be prognostic for the clinical endpoint in order to establish surrogacy.

The different approaches used to quantify the treatment effect on the clinical outcome explained by the surrogate endpoint can be categorized in two groups: (1) analyses based on individual patient data (IPD), and (2) meta-regressions based on summary statistics from the published literature. Although surrogacy assessments on IPD represent the gold standard, at present significant efforts are needed to obtain IPD, and the pay-off for small or poor-quality studies may be low. Issues of ownership and access to data for use in meta-analyses need to be addressed and initiatives to facilitate the use of IPD in meta-analyses set in place.

1.4.1   Validation on Individual Data

The mathematical formulation of a problem that had traditionally been approached by intuition was presented in the landmark paper of Prentice [3], in which a formal definition of a surrogate endpoint was proposed and operational criteria for its validation in the case of a single trial and single surrogate were suggested. According to the definition, a surrogate endpoint is a discrete or continuous, possibly censored, random variable for which a test for the null hypothesis of no treatment effect is also a valid test for the corresponding null hypothesis for the true endpoint. Hence the endpoint is a surrogate for the true endpoint only with respect to the effect of a specific treatment.

Prentice proposed four operational criteria to determine whether a candidate surrogate for a true endpoint fulfils this definition under a specific treatment: (1) the surrogate endpoint is associated with treatment; (2) the true endpoint is associated with treatment; (3) the surrogate and the true endpoints are associated; and (4) given the surrogate endpoint, the treatment and the true endpoint are independent. Popularly, the last criterion is referred to as the *Prentice criterion*.

Freedman, Graubard, and Schatzkin [11] argued that the Prentice criterion is inadequate in the validation of a good surrogate endpoint, since failure to reject the null hypothesis may be due merely to insufficient power (i.e., a low probability of concluding that, given the surrogate, the true endpoint and the treatment are dependent, when this dependency actually exists). Instead, as a measure of the validity of a potential surrogate they proposed using the proportion of the effect of the treatment on the true endpoint that can be explained by the surrogate. A high proportion would indicate that the surrogate is useful. An estimate of the explained proportion is $(\beta - \beta_S)/\beta$ where β and β_S are the estimates of the effect of treatment on the true endpoint, respectively, without and with adjustment for the surrogate.

Several authors have pointed out the drawbacks of this measure. For instance, according to Buyse and Molenberghs [12], the proportion of the treatment effect explained by the surrogate is not truly a proportion, as it can fall out of the [0, 1] interval. As an alternative, they suggested replacing the proportion of treatment effect explained by the surrogate by another set of surrogacy criteria closely related to it: the *relative effect* and the *adjusted association*. The relative effect, defined at the population level, is the ratio between the overall treatment effect on the true endpoint and that on the surrogate endpoint. The adjusted association is the individual-level association between the two endpoints, after accounting for the effect of treatment.

Intuitively, the former is a conversion factor between the treatment effect on the surrogate and that on the primary endpoint. If it were known exactly and the multiplicative relation could be assumed, it could be used to predict the effect of the treatment on the true endpoint based on an observed effect of the treatment on the surrogate. In practice, the relative effect must be estimated, and the precision of that estimate will be relevant for the precision of the prediction.

Generically, the adjusted association is the correlation between the true and surrogate endpoints after adjusting for treatment effect. In a general situation, it is then important to judge whether the correlation is high enough for the surrogate to be trustworthy.

Another line of research has been in the setting of a multi-center trial or a meta-analysis of trials [13]. The association between the two endpoints after adjustment for treatment effect is captured by the squared correlation between the surrogate endpoint and the true endpoint after adjustment for both the trial effects and the treatment effect. This generalization of the adjusted association to the case of several trials is generally referred to as *individual-level surrogacy*. A strong individual-level association implies that the true clinical endpoint can be reliably estimated from the surrogate for individual patients.

Another aspect of surrogacy, measured by the correlation between the effect of treatment on the surrogate and the effect of treatment on the true endpoint, is the *trial-level surrogacy*. A strong trial-level association implies that the effect of treatment on the true clinical endpoint can be reliably estimated from the effect of treatment on the surrogate. With respect to trial-level surrogacy, the concept of a *surrogate threshold effect* (STE) was recently introduced [14]. The STE is defined as the minimum treatment effect on the surrogate required to predict a non-zero treatment effect on the true endpoint in a future trial. If the STE is small, a treatment effect on the true endpoint is likely to be achieved in future studies, in which case the surrogate may be of potential interest. If, in contrast, the STE is large then the surrogate is unlikely to be of practical value. Finally, if the STE cannot be estimated at all, then there is no statistical basis to claims of surrogacy.

More recent research has applied the concepts of causal inference to the assessment of surrogacy. The first approach was that of Robins and Greenland [15]. In their work, the surrogate endpoint is an intermediate variable measured after the baseline covariates and before the outcome. This variable is manipulable and can affect outcome independently of treatment. From a causal viewpoint with respect to surrogacy, it is crucial to be able to formulate appropriate causal pathways in considering the effects of a treatment on a surrogate endpoint and on the true endpoint. This underscore the necessity to improve our understanding of the biological role of surrogates on mechanisms by which treatments of any kind may affect the course of a given disease.

Lassere [16] proposed a formal schema to grade the strength of the relationship between the surrogate endpoint and the true endpoint, based on a weighted evaluation of biological, epidemiological, statistical, clinical trial, and risk-benefit evidence.

1.4.2   Validation on Summary Statistics:
A Meta-analysis Perspective

A meta-analysis evaluates several studies in which a parameter of interest is estimated. In a meta-analysis of clinical trials, the parameter is a measure of the difference in efficacy between the treatment arms. A combination of the estimates is usually achieved based on one of two assumptions (see [17] for a review): (1) methods based on the mathematical assumption that a single common (or "fixed") effect underlies every study in the meta-analysis are referred to as *fixed effect* meta-analyses; (2) methods that assume the use of individual studies to estimate different true treatment effects are referred to as *random-effect* meta-analyses. Another term for such between-study variation is heterogeneity.

There has been a great deal of debate about whether it is better to use a fixed or a random effect meta-analysis. The debate is not about whether the underlying assumption of a fixed effect is likely; rather it is about which is the better trade off: stable robust techniques, with an unlikely underlying assumption, or less stable techniques, based on a somewhat more likely assumption. The random-effects method has long been deemed problematic due to the poor estimation of among-study variance when there is limited information.

In contrast to a simple meta-analysis, combinations of meta-analytic principles with regression ideas (of predicting study effects using study-level covariates) have been developed, namely *meta-regressions* [18]. The outcome variable in a meta-regression analysis is usually a summary statistic, for example, the observed hazard ratio from each trial in case a of time-to-event primary endpoint. Meta-regression aims to relate the size of the effect to one or more study-level characteristics. Its use is appropriate in order to explore sources of heterogeneity even if an initial overall test for heterogeneity [19] is non-significant. Several methods may be applied to estimate fixed and random-effects meta-regression models for the analysis of multiple studies.

The criteria for surrogacy given in the previous section, except those defined at the individual level, may be assessed in summary statistics via meta-regression but several limitations of this approach must be recognized [20]. The associations derived from meta-regressions are observational, although the original studies may have been randomized trials, resulting in a weaker interpretation of the causal relationships than one derived from the original randomized comparisons. This applies particularly when averages of patient characteristics in each study are used as covariates in the regression, since the relationship with patient averages across studies may not be the same as the relationship for patients within studies (ecological bias) [18]. Furthermore, a meta-regression approach will typically be of lower power than an IPD meta-analysis.

The availability of IPD, for both outcomes and covariates, can alleviate some of the problems in meta-regression. In particular, within-trial and between-trial relationships can be more clearly distinguished; in addition, confounding by individual-level covariates can be investigated.

As acknowledged in [14], on the one hand it is important to conduct investigations that allow the evaluation of potential surrogates. These investigations must include information on treatment and on the true clinical endpoint for study participants. On the other hand, it is obviously important to recognize that the large, long, and expensive studies required to fully evaluate potential surrogates are exactly the studies that surrogates were designed to replace. This limitation of surrogacy highlights the importance of continued research involving large clinical trials with true endpoints as well.

1.5   Conclusions

Considering that the number of new therapies entering the market with strong evidence of benefit on survival is not expected to increase, while demands for health cost containment are becoming increasingly pressing, the role of non-validated surrogate endpoints should be carefully reconsidered, both in research and in practice.

In cancer clinical trials, the choice of the primary endpoint should be based on sound biological, pathophysiological, and statistical evaluations to select the best outcome of importance to patients, as well as to determine validity, sensitivity to the study treatment, and feasibility. While in early-phase trials the use of easily measurable surrogate endpoints is unavoidable, quality of life and overall survival should be included as endpoints whenever possible in comparative randomized trials and measured with adequate instruments and length of follow-up.

In the development of evidence-based practice guidelines, the quality of the available evidence should be carefully assessed, with greater attention placed on the a priori importance of the outcomes to be considered in the specific recommendations. The GRADE method represents an excellent approach for this purpose [21]. Positive examples of its application in oncology have been reported [22].

References

1. World Health Organization Mortality estimates by cause, age, and sex for the year 2008 (2011) http://www.who.int/healthinfo/global_burden_disease/en/ Accessed 31 October 2011
2. IOM (Institute of Medicine) (2010) Evaluation of biomarkers and surrogate endpoints in chronic disease. The National Academies Press, Washington, DC
3. Prentice RL (1989) Surrogate endpoints in clinical trials: definition and operational criteria. Stat Med 8:431-440
4. Temple RJ (1995) A regulatory authority's opinion about surrogate endpoints. In: Nimmo WS, Tucker GT (eds) Clinical measurement in drug evaluation. Wiley New York, pp 1-22
5. Biomarkers and surrogate endpoints: preferred definitions and conceptual framework (2001). Clin Pharmacol Ther 69:89-95

6. Shi Q, Sargent DJ (2009) Meta-analysis for the evaluation of surrogate endpoints in cancer clinical trials. Int J Clin Oncol 14:102-111
7. Fleming TR, DeMets DL (1996) Surrogate end points in clinical trials: are we being misled? Ann Intern Med 125:605-613
8. Grimes DA, Schulz KF (2005) Surrogate end points in clinical research: hazardous to your health. Obstet Gynecol 105:1114-1118
9. Johnson JR, Ning YM, Farrell A et al (2011) Accelerated approval of oncology products: the food and drug administration experience. J Natl Cancer Inst 103:636-644
10. Buyse M, Sargent DJ, Grothey A et al (2010) Biomarkers and surrogate end points—the challenge of statistical validation. Nat Rev Clin Oncol 7:309-317
11. Freedman LS, Graubard BI, Schatzkin A (1992) Statistical validation of intermediate endpoints for chronic diseases. Stat Med 11:167-178
12. Buyse M, Molenberghs G (1998) Criteria for the validation of surrogate endpoints in randomized experiments. Biometrics 54:1014-1029
13. Buyse M (2009) Use of meta-analysis for the validation of surrogate endpoints and biomarkers in cancer trials. Cancer J 15:421-425
14. Burzykowski T, Molenberghs G, Buyse M (eds) (2005) The evaluation of surrogate endpoint. Springer, New York
15. Robins JM, Greenland S (1992) Identifiability and exchangeability for direct and indirect effects. Epidemiology 3:143-155
16. Lassere MN (2008) The Biomarker-Surrogacy Evaluation Schema: a review of the biomarker-surrogate literature and a proposal for a criterion-based, quantitative, multidimensional hierarchical levels of evidence schema for evaluating the status of biomarkers as surrogate endpoints. Stat Methods Med Res 17:303-340
17. Sutton AJ, Higgins JP (2008) Recent developments in meta-analysis. Stat Med 27:625-650
18. Thompson SG, Higgins JP (2002) How should meta-regression analyses be undertaken and interpreted? Stat Med 21:1559-1573
19. Higgins JP, Thompson SG, Deeks JJ, Altman DG (2003) Measuring inconsistency in meta-analyses. BMJ 327:557-560
20. Li Z, Meredith MP (2003) Exploring the relationship between surrogates and clinical outcomes: analysis of individual patient data vs. meta-regression on group-level summary statistics. J Biopharm Stat 13:777-792
21. Atkins D, Best D, Briss PA et al, GRADE Working Group (2004) Grading quality of evidence and strength of recommendations. BMJ 328:1490
22. Parmelli E, Papini D, Moja L et al (2010) Updating clinical recommendations for breast, colorectal and lung cancer treatments: an opportunity to improve methodology and clinical relevance. Ann Oncol 22:188-194

Response to Treatment: the Role of Imaging

2

Francesco Sardanelli, Anastasia Esseridou, Angelo S. Del Sole and
Luca M. Sconfienza

2.1   Introduction

Cancer is a major human health problem, both in developing and developed countries. While screening and improved therapies have yielded relevant successes for some forms of cancer—resulting in a 1% annual decline in mortality from all cancers in the USA since 1990—each year, about 7 million people worldwide and 600,000 in the USA continue to die from this disease [1].

Since a completely effective therapy is not available in the large majority of cancers, physicians must evaluate the relative benefit to the patient of a particular treatment. The expected benefit is assessed in terms of a reduction in both the size of the tumor and dissemination of the cancer, i.e., its *response*, also referred to as the degree of *remission* or *regression*. Imaging is an ideal tool with which to evaluate response. In fact, the aim of using imaging as a surrogate biomarker for the response to treatment in oncology is threefold:

1. To obtain a measure of disease extent as a function of treatment that is more objective and reproducible than achieved by considering symptoms or clinical status.
2. To better understand tumor response (based on a comparison of images obtained at baseline and after one or more therapy cycles and with the same imaging technique) at an earlier time than is possible with other biomarkers or with primary end-points, such as overall survival/mortality or disease-specific survival/mortality (see Chapter 1).
3. To reduce, as the combined consequence of points 1 and 2, either the time or the sample size in clinical trials testing new therapies, including drugs, surgery, or imaging-guided interventional procedures.

F. Sardanelli (✉)
Department of Medical Surgical Sciences, University of Milan, Department of Radiology,
IRCCS Policlinico San Donato, San Donato Milanese (Mi), Italy

This unique role of imaging in oncology is related to the differences between general pharmacologic research and oncologic pharmacologic research. In fact, in phase 1 general research, uncontrolled studies mainly address the safety and tolerability of the drug in healthy volunteers whereas in oncologic research the studies are aimed at dose determination and at acquiring preliminary information on the drug's pharmacodynamics in patients, typically those with advanced cancer. In other words, in oncology, proof of concept and dose-finding are anticipated in phase 1 [2].

The need for anticipated information on response to treatment and the crucial role of this type of information for clinical research in oncology explain the efforts to define international criteria for measuring solid tumors and categorizing response as seen on imaging studies. Thus, in 1979–1981 the World Health Organization (WHO) offered a set of criteria for this purpose [3, 4]. These were followed in 2000 by the first version (1.0) of the Response Evaluation Criteria for Solid Tumors (RECIST) [5], and in 2009 by version 1.1 of RECIST [6]. This evolution is not as one would have expected in that there was no linear transition from old to new imaging techniques, or from simple to complex methods. Moreover, the criteria for defining response to oncologic treatment on imaging studies were (and still are) quite conservative in terms of imaging modalities and techniques as well as methods for measuring response. Thus, their evolution was essentially aimed at simplifying measurement procedures.

In this chapter, we describe this evolution and outline the potential role of imaging techniques still not considered by these formalized criteria. In this context, we discuss oncologic imaging as a tool to evaluate the response to treatment and thus as a relevant example of *quantitative imaging*, which is probably the most tremendous challenge for the future of radiology.

2.2   WHO Criteria

Criteria issued by the WHO 30 years ago [3, 4] were based on an intuitive concept for two-dimensional (2D) imaging such as computed tomography (CT): multiplying the longest diameter of a cancer lesion by its largest perpendicular diameter, i.e., to obtain its *cross-product*. Tumor response was classified into one of four categories according to the percentage change in cross-product at follow-up compared with baseline, as follows:

$$[(\text{Cross-product}_{\text{Follow-up}} - \text{Cross-product}_{\text{Baseline}})/\text{Cross-product}_{\text{Baseline}}] \times 100$$

In case of multiple lesions in an individual patient, cross-products were summed. The four categories for tumor response were as follows:
- *Complete response* (CR): in case of tumor disappearance.
- *Partial response* (PR): in case of a cross-product decrease ≥ 50%.
- *Progressive disease* (PD): in case of a cross-product increase ≥ 25%.
- *Stable disease* (SD): when the change in the cross-product cannot be

categorized as CR, PR, or PD.

An interval of at least 4 weeks was required for confirming the CR or PR categories. These criteria were used in clinical trials for more than 20 years. However, neither the imaging modalities to be used nor the number and minimal size of the lesions to be measured were defined. These limitations were associated with the use of imaging techniques intrinsically burdened by lower reproducibility or with the evaluation of lesions too small to ensure reproducibility. Moreover, the cutoff for PD (cross-product increase ≥ 25%) was relatively low, leading to its possible overestimation and an incorrect evaluation of the inefficacy of an effective treatment. Consequently, over two decades, standardization was complicated by numerous proposed modifications up until 2000, when new internationally accepted criteria were established.

2.3   RECIST 1.0

In 2000, the European Organization for Research and Treatment of Cancer and the National Cancer Institutes of the USA and Canada introduced the RECIST criteria, version 1.0 [5].

First, RECIST moved from 2D to one-dimensional (1D) measurements. In fact, the axial cross-product was abandoned and the evaluation of tumor response was now based only on a variation of the longest axial diameter. Again, measurements of multiple lesions were summed. Moreover, RECIST 1.0 established a series of new rules:

- Use of CT or magnetic resonance imaging (MRI).
- Definition of a maximum of 10 *target lesions* in total (maximum 5 per organ).
- A minimum size for the target lesion (10 mm for spiral CT; 20 mm for non-spiral CT or MRI).

Notably, target lesions had to be chosen based not only on their size but also on their characteristics, thus allowing for their reproducible measurement (well-defined margins, location with reduced movement artifacts, etc.). *Non-target lesions* were defined as non-measurable lesions and measurable lesions not defined as the target. The response categories were as follows:

1. *Complete response* (CR): in case of disappearance of all target and non-target lesions.
2. *Partial response* (PR): in case of a ≥ 30% decrease in the longest diameter (instead of the ≥ 50% of the WHO criteria for the cross-product) and/or persistence of non-target lesions.
3. *Progressive disease* (PD): in case of a ≥ 20% increase in the longest diameter of the target lesions (instead of the ≥ 25% of the WHO criteria for the cross-product), the appearance of one or more new lesions, or unequivocal progression of already existing non-target lesions.
4. *Stable disease* (SD): when the case cannot be categorized as CR, PR, or PD
   The CR and PR categories needed to be confirmed after at least 28 days.

This striking change in methods, from 2D to 1D measurement, even if based on results in more than 4,000 patients in 14 clinical trials [5], is quite counterintuitive. Was it a step backward? Aren't two (dimensions) obviously better than one? The rational basis for this approach is the realistic comparison between a long cigar and a rugby ball: they might have the same longest diameter but the volume of the latter is much greater. Thus, while volume – and thus a three-dimensional (3D) measurement – should be the best, at least 2D should be better than 1D. *However, the preference for 2D instead of 1D works only if the reproducibility of the two lengths measured to obtain the area, or cross-product, is relatively high.*

Here is a simple example. You have a tumor image on a CT slice at baseline and you determine that it measures 3×4 cm; yielding, according to WHO criteria, a cross-product of 12 cm^2. At follow-up, the tumor has not changed but the exam is evaluated by a younger colleague who tends to overestimate the longest diameter by 15% in length compared to your own measurements (notably, an 85% inter-observer reproducibility is indeed acceptable). This colleague measures tumor dimensions of 3.45×4.6 cm, i.e., a cross-product of 15.87 cm^2. The cross-product indicates an increase in tumor size (in cm^2) of $(15.87 – 12.00)/12 = 0.32$. According to the WHO criteria, a 32% cross-product increase, i.e., $\geq 25\%$, should be reported as PD, although in reality the size of the tumor is unchanged and the correct report would be SD. With RECIST 1.0, the same error in measurement gives an increase (in cm) of $(4.6 – 4.0)/4.0 = 0.15$. A 15% increase in the longest diameter is below the new cutoff for PD ($\geq 20\%$); thus, the measurement error does not influence the reported RECIST 1.0 category: SD. One should note that this is not simply due to the use of 1D instead of 2D, but also to the higher cutoff for PD in RECIST 1.0. In fact, assuming a spherical tumor volume, a 25% increase in the 2D cross-product is equal to a 40% increase in the 3D volume, while a 20% 1D increase in the longest diameter is equal to a 44% 2D increase in the cross-product and to a 73% increase in 3D volume [1]. This implies that the time to PD measured using RECIST 1.0 is longer than that measured with the WHO criteria, showing that these cutoffs are somewhat arbitrary even though they are based on data obtained from thousands of patients enrolled in clinical trials.

Moreover, if a trial has adopted WHO at its beginning, the same method must be used up to its conclusion (the same is valid for RECIST 1.0 vs. RECIST 1.1). For long trials, this golden rule is necessarily challenged by technological developments. In other words, even though measurements might be unchanged, the imaging equipment certainly has, allowing for higher diagnostic performance, at least at the lower level of efficacy, i.e., so-called technical performance [7]. This was the case when 16-slice CT was replaced by ≥ 64-slice machines, or, in MRI, as the number of channels increased first to 16, then to 32, 64, and more (or the field strength increased from 1.5 to 3 T). The effect is a kind of *technological bias* that hampers reliable longitudinal comparisons in clinical trials. It is the downside of technological development, which for imaging specialists provides not only extraordinary opportunities but also problems, especially when the speed of technological change is greater than that needed to obtain scientific evidence of at least a diagnostic benefit for patients from the new technology [8].

2.4   RECIST 1.1

In 2009, almost 10 years after the introduction of RECIST 1.0, new RECIST criteria (version 1.1) were proposed [6] on the basis of results obtained for over 18,000 potential target lesions in over 6,500 patients in 16 trials. Again, the aim was to standardize and simplify but also to consider issues not taken into account in the previous version; thus:

1. The number of target lesions was reduced from 10 to 5 (maximum 2 per organ) (Fig. 2.1).
2. The minimum size of target lesions was set at ≥ 10 mm for spiral CT or MRI, ≥ 20 mm for chest X-ray.
3. The 1D longest diameter of the tumors was included.
4. The 1D longest short-axis diameter for lymph nodes was also included. Lymph nodes with a short axis ≥ 10 mm are considered as positive for cancer involvement, but only those with a short axis ≥ 15 mm are amenable for measurement as target lesions, as single organs; lymph nodes ≥ 10 mm and < 15 mm in diameter are considered as non-target lesions. (Fig. 2.2).
5. The condition of complete recovery (CR) was defined not only as the disappearance of all target lesions but also the reduction of all (target or non-target) lymph nodes to < 10 mm (short axis).
6. The slice thickness at CT or MRI had to be no more than one half of the size of the target lesion at its smallest diameter (to avoid relevant partial volume effects).
7. Contrast-enhanced CT or MRI and use of the same or similar technical parameters as at baseline or previous follow-up were recommended (for higher reproducibility).
8. To declare a condition of progressive disease (PD) in absence of new lesions, an increase in the sum of the longest diameters of target lesions ≥ 20%

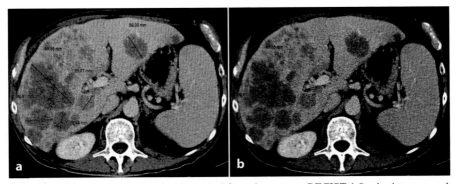

Fig. 2.1 A 65-year-old male previously treated for colon cancer. RECIST 1.0 criteria were used to measure five liver metastases as target lesions (**a**); according to the RECIST 1.1 criteria, only the two largest metastases are measured as target lesions (**b**)

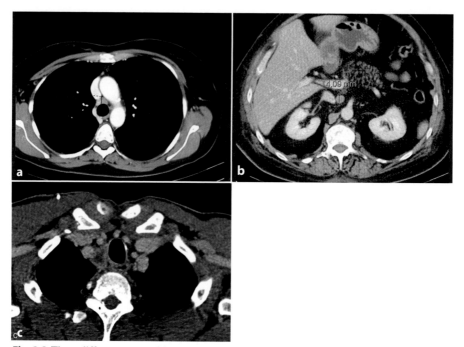

Fig. 2.2 Three different cases of lymph node measurements in oncology patients. **a** Pretracheal lymph node with a short axis of 10 mm in a patient with cancer at the esophageal-gastric junction; the lymph node is positive for metastatic involvement but cannot be considered as a target lesion. **b** A retroperitoneal lymph node, located close to the inferior vena cava in a patient with colon cancer; the short axis is > 14 mm but not ≥ 15 mm: it is positive for metastatic involvement but cannot be considered as a target lesion. **c** A partially necrotic paratracheal lymph node in the upper mediastinum in a patient with cancer at the middle portion of the esophagus; it can be considered as a target lesion, its short axis being > 17 mm

alone is not sufficient if the absolute increase in this sum is lower than 5 mm. This prevents small errors in lesion diameter measurements from determining a PD diagnosis, which is important especially in the follow-up of small residual disease, when a minimal increase due only to measurement variability could be wrongly judged as PD.

9. Information obtained with ^{18}F-fluorodeoxyglucose (^{18}F-FDG) positron emission tomography (PET) is taken into account in the detection of new lesions or to confirm CR or PD (Fig. 2.3).

The rules and criteria for categorizing tumor response according to RECIST 1.1 are summarized in Table 2.1. Importantly, specific rules have to be applied to consider a new lesion, seen on PET, as evidence of PD. In this case, contrast-enhanced CT is used as the confirming modality (see note "b" in Table 2.1).

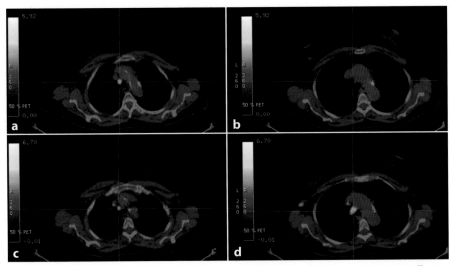

Fig. 2.3 ^{18}F-FDG PET CT performed in a 76-year-old female in whom breast cancer was discovered in 2000. She underwent surgery, followed by radiation therapy, chemotherapy, and hormonal therapy. **a, b** In July 2011, a metastasis in a paratracheal lymph node was detected (SUVmax 6.4). **c** After chemotherapy, in December 2011, ^{18}F-FDG PET CT showed persistent metabolic activity in this metastasis (SUVmax 5.8). **d** Moreover, two additional metastases (another large paratracheal lymph node and a deep lymph node in the right axilla) were detected, resulting in progressive disease. Note the absence of these two lesions in July 2011 (**b**)

Note that the reduction from ten to five target lesions implies a 70% reduction in measurements, without reducing the amount of information on disease evolution [9] while increasing the reproducibility in declaring PD, as shown for patients with non-small-cell lung cancer [10]. Moreover, the use of RECIST 1.1 instead of RECIST 1.0 criteria probably reduces the time for image analysis by radiologists involved in oncology clinical trials by about one-third. In fact, lesion measurement accounts for only part of the time needed for the careful evaluation of a follow-up contrast-enhanced body CT and comparison with baseline images.

The limitations of the RECIST criteria are evident, as evidenced by the many other methods proposed for specific oncological indications, especially liver neoplasms (see Chapters 3 and 9). In 2001, the European Association for the Study of the Liver (EASL) [11] proposed a method for evaluating hepatocellular carcinoma (HCC) response based on the 2D evaluation of viable residual/necrosis tumor (see Chapter 9). In 2004, Choi and coworkers [12] proposed a combination of size and/or density for evaluating the response of gastrointestinal stromal tumors (GISTs) to imatinib mesylate (see Chapter 3). More recently, several other methods aimed at evaluating the response of HCC to treatment have been proposed, combining viable/necrotic tumor size with distinctions of target/non-target/new lesions or tumor markers levels, such as

Table 2.1 Rules and criteria for categorizing tumor response according to RECIST 1.1

Rules	
Imaging modalities	Contrast-enhanced CT (or MRI for abdominal studies) using ≤ 5-mm slice thicknes (chest x-ray only for pulmonary lesions ≥ 20 mm) ^{18}F-FDG PET (detection of new lesions or confirmation of CR or PD)[a]
Technical parameters	Same or similar between baseline and follow-up studies Slice thickness with a maximum one half of the size of the smallest target lesion
Target lesions	Measurable lesions (longest axial diameter ≥ 10 mm with detectable margins)
Number of target lesions	5 (maximum 2 per organ)
Minimum size of target lesions	Not less than 10 mm on CT or MRI
Size measurement of target lesions	Tumors: 1D longest diameter Lymph nodes: longest short axis diameter (positive when ≥ 10 mm; target lesions only when ≥ 15 mm)
Non-target lesions	Potentially target lesions other than 5 in total or 2 per organ Non-measurable lesions: lesions with axial longest diameter < 10 mm; skeletal metastases without well detectable soft-tissue component; pleural effusion and ascites; lymphangitic or leptomeningeal tumor diffusion; inflammatory breast cancer; cystic or necrotic tumor lesions; lesions inside a body part treated with radiation therapy
Criteria for tumor response	
Complete response (CR)	Disappearance of all target lesions
	AND: Reduction of all (target and non-target) lymph nodes to <10 mm in short axis AND: No new lesions[a]
Partial response (PR)	Target lesions: decrease in the sum of longest diameters ≥ 30%
	AND: Disappearance or persistence of already existing non-target lesions[b] AND: No new lesions[a]
Stable disease (SD)	All conditions not classifiable as CR, PR, or PD
Progressive disease (PD)	Increase in the sum of longest diameters of target lesions ≥ 5 mm (absolute) AND ≥ 20% (relative to baseline) OR: One or more new lesions[a] OR: Unequivocal progression of already existing non-target lesions[b]

[a]A new lesion on a follow-up ^{18}F-FDG PET scan should be evaluated as follows:
If not present at a previous PET scan, PD is declared.
In the absence of a baseline/previous PET scan, if the new lesion on PET is confirmed at CT, declare PD, if not confirmed, additional CT scans are needed to decide whether or not to declare PD.
If the lesion corresponds to one detectable on a previous CT and it has not progressed at follow-up CT, PD should not be declared.
[b]Modest increase in the size of non-target lesions cannot justify declaring PD.

the mRECIST criteria of the American Association for the Study of Liver [13] and the RECICL criteria of the Liver Cancer Study Group of Japan [14].

In general, purely dimensional criteria, such as those of the WHO and RECIST 1.1 guidelines, despite the great advantage they offer in terms of standardization and reproducibility, are extremely conservative compared to the therapeutic developments and, especially, to the technological evolution in imaging capability.

2.5   CT Beyond Diameters: Density, Perfusion, and the 3D (Volume) Challenge

CT has evolved rapidly in the last decade. Multi-slice acquisition established 16- and 64-slice machines as the new standards, and machines with > 64 slices as advanced units. The latter were initially applied in cardiac imaging but have now been extended to other indications. Moreover, dual-source/energy approaches are furthering diagnostic possibilities, including for tumor response evaluation [15].

Nonetheless, CT fundamentally remains a method in which information is derived from electronic density measurements. While this has been discarded by the standardized WHO and RECIST methods, density was added as a relevant parameter in a number of proposals. The method of Choi et al. for GISTs [12] and the above-mentioned methods for HCC response [11, 13, 14] are typical examples. A paradoxical increase in tumor size after treatment due to hemorrhage or necrosis is one of several typical issues not considered in the RECIST guidelines [16]. Lung cancer cavitation after chemotherapy poses similar problems in that the total lesion volume may be more or less unchanged while that of the tumor tissue is greatly reduced (see Chapter 7). Crabb et al. [17], who continue to use the 1D measurement method, proposed subtracting the longest diameter of the cavity from the longest diameter of the mass.

A further approach to contrast-enhanced CT for tumor response evaluation has come from *perfusion* studies, i.e., by fast repetition of volume acquisition after intravenous administration of iodinated contrast agent, allowing for the extraction of dynamic parameters useful in the evaluation of tumor tissue [18]. Applications to tumor response have been reported in the literature, in particular for studies of liver and colorectal cancers [19, 20]. Importantly, recent perfusion CT (and MRI) studies have the advantage of not being limited to one or a few slices, instead encompassing the whole tumor volume, thereby allowing for volumetric perfusion evaluations. Thus, there has been a shift from 1D or 2D to 3D imaging, and even four-dimensional (4D) if the time dimension is considered as well.

However, while, today, 3D volumetric assessment is possible using modern multislice CT units (as well as MRI and 3D ultrasound), the geometric issues deserve to be carefully considered. Here the challenge is good reproducibility, which becomes increasingly difficult. In fact, the addition of a third dimension to volumetric assessment increases the error.

Let us to return to the simple example presented in Sect. 2.3. Evaluation of the same 3×4 cm lesion by two readers had an 85% reproducibility, based on the difference of 15% using 1D and 32% using 2D methods. What happens using 3D? By simply adding the third dimension, we increase the error percentage. Thus, for a mass of $3 \times 4 \times 3$ cm (calculating the volume as area by height, to maintain the similarity with the cross-product), if the first reader correctly measures only 36 cm^3, the measurements determined by the second reader would be $3.45 \times 4.6 \times 3.45 = 54.7515$ cm^3, corresponding to a false increase of about 19/36 cm^3, equal to 53%. Is the take-home lesson then: the greater the number of dimensions used, the lower the reproducibility of the measurement? Yes, it is simple Euclidean geometry, even though it remains counterintuitive, as demonstrated by the usual reporting of two, sometimes three dimensions for masses or nodules in many organs on ultrasound (US), CT, or MRI.

However, this line of reasoning has a weak point: since the tumor is a 3D object, the more dimensions used, the closer one is to reality. The problem is that as dimensions are added, the reproducibility must be correspondingly higher. In other words, areas or volumes cannot be reliably represented by multiple 1D diameters; rather, measurements of areas and volumes require other tools, i.e., dedicated software. Our own experience is with growing region segmentation software (based on pixel thresholding) for both lesion area measurement [21] and the automatic definition of new lesions [22], as evaluated in longitudinal trials on multiple sclerosis using MRI as the imaging modality, but there are similar CT-based methods for use in determining liver tumor response after trans-arterial chemoembolization [23]. This is a promising field of research requiring careful evaluation not only of intra- and inter-observer reproducibility, but also of inter-study reproducibility [2]. As a matter of fact, although fully automatic (unsupervised) tumor segmentation methods are being reported, such as the recent personal experience for breast MRI [24], the majority of these approaches are semi-automatic and therefore still need human intervention. Furthermore, all these methods must be fully verified to be sufficiently reproducible.

2.6   Magnetic Resonance Imaging and More…

"MR imaging belongs to the most rapidly evolving techniques of contemporary clinical medicine – for good or bad, this jeopardizes attempts to standardize the modality. Accordingly, prescribing a detailed imaging protocol would probably be futile because such a protocol would be outdated the very day of its publication" [25]. This sentence by Cristiane K. Khul, related to breast MRI, is valid for the entire spectrum of MRI techniques for tumor response evaluation. In fact, in this setting MRI allows for a number of technical possibilities. We mention only those commonly available for standard MRI units

used in clinical practice:
1. Standard T1- and T2-weighted imaging.
2. Dynamic contrast-enhanced (DCE) imaging.
3. Contrast-enhanced T2*-weighted perfusion studies.
4. Diffusion-weighted imaging (DWI).
5. ^{1}H (proton) MR spectroscopy (MRS).

As noted above, rapid technological evolution limits complete standardization.

Mathematical modeling [26] is used for extracting the following parameters from DCE-MRI:
1. K^{trans} = rate of contrast agent transfer from the blood to the interstitium.
2. k_{ep} = rate of contrast agent transfer from the interstitium to the blood (backflow).
3. fpV = fraction of plasma volume.
4. V_e = extravascular volume.

However, DCE-MRI is sufficiently robust to be used for clinical patient care and can be implemented in multicenter clinical trials evaluating tumor response. The technical requirements and range of acceptable sequence parameters can be defined such that they are respected by all the enrolling centers.

What is relatively unexpected is that CT is usually preferred to MRI in clinical oncologic evaluation and that, also for clinical trials, the tremendous potential of MRI is largely underexploited. This could be due to several factors, including: the lower availability of MRI units; the reduced familiarity with MRI of oncologists, radiation therapists, and other physicians of the cancer team; the higher cost; and, last but not least, the limited involvement of radiologists in decision-making committees for oncologic research. This aspect is also implied in the low profile of radiologists in the authorship of secondary studies (meta-analyses, guidelines, etc.) concerning the diagnostic performance of imaging techniques [27]: Indeed, from 2001 to 2010, in over 1,000 papers evaluated, a radiologist (or a nuclear medicine physician) was the first author in only 16%, the second author in only 15%, and the senior (last) author in only 13%.

Importantly, non-contrast MRI techniques are playing an increasingly important role in oncological imaging (Fig. 2.4). On the one hand, DWI has been shown to perform better than contrast-enhanced dynamic studies in evaluating residual breast cancer after neoadjuvant chemotherapy [28], with a similar sensitivity (0.97 vs. 0.93) but a significantly better specificity (0.89 vs. 0.56). Breast DWI suffers from false-positives less often than DCE imaging in evaluating tumor response (see Chapter 6). The applications of DWI are expanding to many forms of cancer, allowing for repeatable, low-cost, and non-invasive approaches during treatment. Notably, DWI enables the observer to produce a region-of-interest (ROI)-based lesion quantification in terms of apparent diffusion coefficient (ADC), an indicator of tumor response, suggested by an early ADC increase after treatment [29, 30].On the other hand, whole-body DWI is a potential alternative to PET for oncologic staging [31].

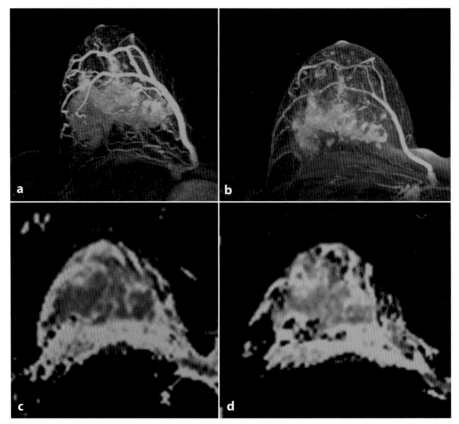

Fig. 2.4 A locally advanced invasive ductal cancer in the right breast of a 50-year-old woman. Contrast-enhanced MRI (maximum intensity projection) shows a huge enhancing mass and increased whole-breast vascularity before neoadjuvant chemotherapy (NAC) (**a**) and reduced mass vascularity after NAC (**b**). Diffusion-weighted MRI (maps of apparent diffusion coefficient) shows the restricted diffusion of the mass (*dark gray*) before NAC (**c**) and a relative diffusion increase (*middle gray*) of the reduced mass after NAC (**d**)

Especially as an early predictor of response, MRS may have a more intriguing potential [32-34]. This is due to its peculiar insight into cell metabolism, based on its ability to detect and quantify choline-containing compounds in tumors [35]. The choline peak can be evaluated in vivo also at only 1.5 Tesla, as shown in personal experiences for breast [36] and ovarian [37] cancers. However, it should be emphasized that MRS is still an investigational tool whose use continues to be limited due to the significantly prolonged acquisition time and the frequent artifacts resulting from patient movements. Importantly, in MRS, post-processing is relatively complex as well as time-consuming, especially if multi-voxel, chemical shift imaging 3D sequences are used. Thus, at the present time, MRS cannot be proposed as an "imaging" tool for day-by-day clinical practice or large multicenter trials. This is not the case with DWI, which has a short acquisition time and relatively simpler post-processing.

2.7   Ultrasonography

Traditionally, US has been excluded from the imaging modalities used to assess tumor response, given its low reproducibility and high operator dependence. In fact, although the measurement of a single known lesion using US could be reproducible, US evaluation is performed in real-time and complete examinations cannot be provided for an independent review at later stages. Moreover, especially in the presence of hepatic or abdominal nodules, some anatomic regions may not be adequately evaluated if the bowel overlies the organ and the US beam cannot penetrate the gas contained therein. Recently developed US techniques, such as tissue harmonic imaging, have improved the diagnostic capabilities of conventional B-mode imaging. However, the ability of US to demonstrate tumor necrosis within a nodule can be severely limited by the altered transonic impedance produced by collateral factors, such as intra-tumor hemorrhage during sorafenib therapy. Color and power Doppler US provide functional data on tumor vasculature (e.g., velocity, spectral profiles, resistivity index), allowing for a global evaluation of tumor macrovasculature. However, these tools cannot be used to monitor early treatment response, as they are unable to detect the microvasculature and are inadequate to evaluate neo-angiogenesis. Notably, RECIST 1.1 criteria [6] recommend CT or MRI confirmation of any unknown US-detected lesion seen during the course of a clinical study.

Specifically designed contrast agents (such as sulfur hexafluoride contained in phospholipid-coated microbubbles or perfluorobutane gas microspheres stabilized by a membrane of hydrogenated egg phosphatidyl serine) allow these limitations to be partially overcome (Fig. 2.5). A great advantage of these contrast agents is that they are merely intravascular. Also, microbubbles are extremely small (~3 μm) because they need to easily pass the pulmonary filter. They enable the detection of vessels as narrow as 40 μm in diameter. Accordingly, contrast-enhanced US (CEUS) offers a precise evaluation of changes in tumor microvessel density. In addition, US contrast agents are as effective as CT or MRI agents in the detection of residual active tumor tissue within the necrotic area induced by treatment [38]. CEUS also has been successfully used to monitor thermal ablation procedures either during or after treatment, being able to detect the presence of remnant viable cancer tissue [39]. In the liver, CEUS has been demonstrated to be effective in the follow-up of lesions that were undetectable on B-mode US studies after chemotherapy.

The real-time evaluation of contrast behavior (dynamic-CEUS, DCE-US) determines contrast flow parameters (e.g., peak enhancement, time-to-peak intensity, mean transit time) and can therefore be used to assess a very early response to treatment. Additional applications are the evaluation of tumor response to anti-angiogenic drugs, such as sorafenib or bevacizumab [40, 41]. Interestingly, a rich pre-treatment vascularization was shown to positively correlate with a good response. Response to treatment at early stages can be predicted based on changes in vascularization, even in the absence of changes in tumor volume [38].

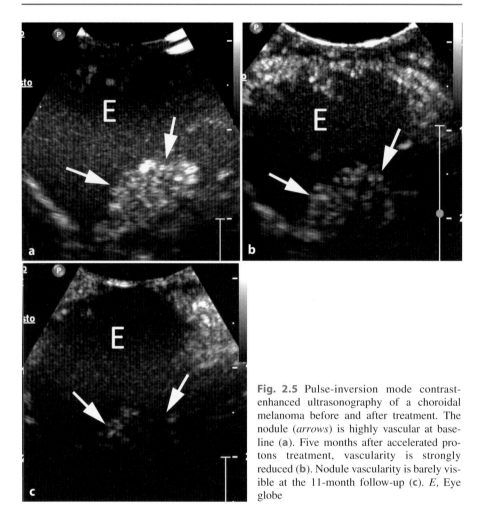

Fig. 2.5 Pulse-inversion mode contrast-enhanced ultrasonography of a choroidal melanoma before and after treatment. The nodule (*arrows*) is highly vascular at baseline (**a**). Five months after accelerated protons treatment, vascularity is strongly reduced (**b**). Nodule vascularity is barely visible at the 11-month follow-up (**c**). *E,* Eye globe

Recently, specific software has been developed to increase the diagnostic potential of DCE-US [42]. These systems can derive time-intensity curves from a continuous real-time scanning. Lesion tracking and movement compensation tools are employed to reduce artifact occurrence, thus potentially increasing precision and objectivity. However, the reproducibility of DCE-US with respect to tumor treatment outcome has yet to be reported and the quantification software suffers from limitations. The current trend is to measure only relative perfusion (perfusion in the lesion compared to the surrounding healthy parenchyma), as absolute perfusion is not considered to be a reliable parameter. Also, dynamic curves can be affected by the inhomogeneity of the US field and by microbubble destruction, both of which can occur during focus adjustments made to allow for continuous real-time scanning.

Recent technological developments have modified the traditional secondary role of US in tumor response evaluation, but not all the associated problems have been solved. However, specific fields are now defined, especially for DCE-US for liver tumors. Radiologists should promote the establishment of research trials aimed at testing the reproducibility of new US techniques and comparing the diagnostic performance of US with that of CT or MRI in the setting of tumor response evaluation.

2.8   Positron Emission Tomography

As reported in Sect. 2.4, the 2009 RECIST 1.1 criteria [6] finally included ^{18}F-FDG PET as an imaging modality for detecting/excluding new lesions or confirming CR or PD. Considering that PET entered clinical practice in 1979-1980 – that is, about 30 years before worldwide acceptance of radionuclide tomographic imaging in clinical trials for the treatment of solid tumors – this clearly demonstrates the conservative thinking in clinical oncology. But there are reasons for this cautiousness: essentially, the need for a high level of standardization and reproducibility for any test, including those based on imaging, that will be used in multicenter clinical trials. Nevertheless, this seems to be an overly long delay, especially after the advent of hybrid PET/CT imaging in 1999-2000, which offered a novel combination of functional/molecular information (from PET) and anatomic/topographic resolution (from CT). PET is certainly the most striking imaging innovation in oncology in recent decades. Its unique ability to visualize disease-related molecular and biological characteristics makes PET a *must* for cancer centers worldwide.

Many tumor-seeking radiopharmaceuticals are now available, but ^{18}F-FDG accounts for 90% of the PET exams performed worldwide [43]. It is analogous to glucose in its competition for uptake by glucose transporters (GLUT) and as a substrate for phosphorylation. A radioactive fluorine molecule is located in the 2 position of glucose. The key feature of ^{18}F-FDG-6-P is that it is not a substrate for further metabolism, unlike glucose-6-phosphate. Consequently, it accumulates in tissues in proportion to the glucose metabolic rate. Although complete trapping of this tracer cannot be achieved, images acquired between 40 and 60 min after its intravenous injection accurately reflect the glycolytic activity of body tissues. Increased glucose consumption is characteristic of most tumor cells and is partially related to their overexpression of GLUT-1 and increased hexokinase activity [44]. A rather strong relationship between ^{18}F-FDG uptake and cancer cell number has been shown in a number of studies [45-47]. In the setting of cancer staging, PET/CT is superior to other imaging modalities for most tumor types. It was shown to up-stage about 40% of lymphomas and to change the management of 30% of patients with non-small-cell lung cancers (mainly preventing unnecessary surgery) and 35% of those with colorectal cancer. In addition, its role in post-treatment evaluation is clinically relevant for many cancers, in particular for lymphoma, colorectal cancer, and tumors of the head/neck, breast, esophagus, pancreas, and cervix, as well as for sarcomas and melanomas [43].

Since ^{18}F-FDG uptake is not confined to tumor cells and may also be seen in physiological conditions (brown fat, colonic and gynecologic activity), inflammatory cells, and macrophages, the specificity of PET is limited, as it is not always possible to differentiate tumor from focal infection, granulomatous lesions, or macrophage infiltration of necrotic tissue [48]. ^{18}F-FDG uptake may also be overestimated in tumors with an inflammatory component or, more often, because of radiation-mediated inflammatory processes (that may persist for weeks to months). Many other factors influence the apparent post-therapeutic alterations in tumor ^{18}F-FDG uptake, including a change in lesion size, perfusion, cell number, or proliferative activity, tumor glucose utilization, tumor heterogeneity, and reversible cell damage. Clinical PET studies of tumor response have taken a pragmatic approach, relating observed changes in tumor ^{18}F-FDG uptake to clinical outcome and pathologic findings, the latter being determined in the case of preoperative (radio-) chemotherapy [49].

Absolute quantification of glycolytic metabolism can be theoretically obtained with rigorous compartmental modeling of ^{18}F-FDG kinetics, for example, by fitting tissue time-activity curves to a two- or three-compartment model, using an arterial input function and non-linear regression techniques to determine the metabolic rate of glucose in moles/min/ml. However, the difficulties in developing robust tracer kinetic models applicable to heterogeneous tumor masses and the limited spatial resolution intrinsic to PET instrumentation make it very difficult to achieve absolute quantitative measurement of glycolysis in tumors on the basis of ^{18}F-FDG uptake. Therefore, various surrogate semi-quantitative methods have been developed to standardize tracer uptake measures. The most widely used are the *tumor-to-normal tissue ratio* (T/N ratio) and the *standardized uptake value* (SUV).

The T/N ratio compares tumor activity with the activity of normal tissues. It does not require accurate quantitative determination of tissue activity nor is it affected by the injected dose, patient body weight, or blood glucose level. It is also not sensitive to changes in the distribution of tracer to other tissues, as may occur with extravasation of injected tracer or a decrease in renal excretion. A change in the T/N ratio is similar to a change in visual contrast and can occur in response to alterations in normal tissue uptake in the absence of altered tumor activity. Also, it may be difficult to select an appropriate adjacent normal reference site, particularly in the abdomen and pelvis, where there is marked variation in uptake both between studies and between patients. Although some authors have demonstrated the usefulness of the T/N ratio in selected cases, the drawbacks are its low reproducibility and operator-dependence [50].

SUV is defined as the tissue concentration of tracer, as measured by a PET scanner, divided by the injected activity divided by body weight. It is equivalent to the ratio between the amount of ^{18}F-FDG that accumulates in a lesion and the amount of tracer that would eventually be present in the same region if the

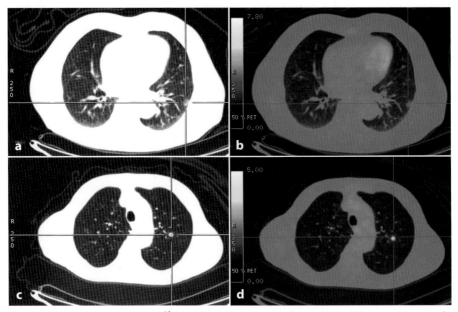

Fig. 2.6 SUV$_{max}$ measurement of ^{18}F-FDG uptake in lung nodules of two different patients. **a, b** The SUV$_{max}$ measured in a ground-glass lesion of the left lung was only 1.03, which is considered not significant for cancer. **c, d** A SUV$_{max}$ of 3.71 was considered suspicious for malignant disease

tracer was homogeneously distributed in the body. It is expressed as:

$$SUV = (Radioactivity\ in\ tissue/Weight\ of\ tissue)/(Injected\ radioactivity/Weight\ of\ patient)$$

From a practical point of view, an SUV > 1 implies tracer accumulation due to metabolic activity, while 1 is the background value due to unspecific tracer distribution (Fig. 2.6). To overcome falsely high SUVs in obese patients, the data are normalized using patient lean body mass (lbm) instead of body weight (SUV$_{lbm}$) [51].

A fundamental biological question underlying the choice of ROI for SUV analysis is whether the total tumor volume or the maximally metabolically active portion of the tumor is most important. Intuitively, the answer would be both; however, insight into stem cell biology suggests that the most critically important parts of tumors are their most aggressive portions, which may not be the entire tumor. This is commonly applied in SUV analysis, as this value is frequently obtained from pixels with SUV$_{max}$ and, although not usually determined in this way, it could be considered as a single-pixel ROI. For SUV$_{max}$ to be used routinely in the assessment of response to treatment, its performance characteristics should be well understood, including its reproducibility versus other approaches. Nonetheless, SUV$_{max}$ is the simplest method, with low interobserver variability, widespread use, and demonstrated effectiveness in differentiating malignancies from benign diseases [49].

Methods for determining total lesion glycolysis are still evolving. The choice of a threshold based on a single maximal pixel value in the tumor carries with it the variability inherent in determining a single-pixel value and is driven by that value. The use of thresholds related to background activity is one approach that has been applied to avoid the uncertainty of SUV_{max}. Other approaches include the determination of lesion volume not from PET but from the CT component of PET/CT; regardless of the method, these effects should be carefully considered when PET is used for radiotherapy planning or in the evaluation of effect of treatment [52].

Compared with morphological markers, biological/functional markers are subject to a higher inter- and intra-individual variability. Guidelines are available to assure that key parameters (physical activity, metabolic state, activity dose, hydration, stimulation of diuresis, medication, comfortable surroundings, and time point of imaging) are standardized [53]. The plasma glucose level at the time of the study has a major effect on ^{18}F-FDG distribution, and intrasubject variations in plasma glucose can have significant effects on measured SUVs. Precautions must be taken to assure that this variable is carefully monitored, both before tracer injection at baseline exam and after treatment.

Serial ^{18}F-FDG PET imaging, like any other surrogate biomarker, can be used for treatment evaluation in two ways: prediction (to potentially switch to a more effective treatment regimen) and assessment of tumor response (e.g., when treatment failure will lead to second-line therapy in addition to the full initial course). While the final response may be evaluated with a single PET study, response prediction usually requires pre-/post-treatment comparison scans.

As ^{18}F-FDG uptake reflects cancer cell number, one would expect an association between a decline in tumor uptake and a loss of viable cancer cells, and between increased tumor glucose use and volume of tumor cells and disease progression. Cancers are usually detected when they reach a minimum size of 10–100 g (about 10^{10}–10^{11} cells). With current PET systems, the limit of resolution ranges between 4 and 10 mm, i.e. a tumor size of 0.1–0.5 to 1.0 g (or 10^8–10^9 cells). It follows that PET can measure only the first 2 logs of tumor cell kill, depending on the initial size of the tumor. Thus, a negative PET scan at the end of therapy can mean either that there are no cancer cells present or that up to 10^7 cells are still alive, even though either one typically suggests a good prognosis. Conversely, in the absence of inflammation, a positive ^{18}F-FDG PET scan at the end of treatment is usually a sign of residual tumor. Notably, for certain non-cytotoxic agents, PET scans normalize much more quickly than anatomic changes, thus providing a better early prediction of outcome [9].

The future perspectives of PET in oncologic imaging are based on the potential use of newer tracers targeting specific biological processes, such as proliferation ([18]F- fluorothymidine [^{18}F-FLT]), angiogenesis (^{18}F-galacto-arginine-glycine-aspartic acid [^{18}F-RGD]), apoptosis (Annexin-V), and hypoxia (^{18}F-fluoromisonidazole [^{18}F-FMISO], ^{18}F-fluoroazomycin arabinoside [^{18}F-FAZA]) [49]. As key processes in oncogenesis, these imaging targets are expected to provide meaningful information for the selection and monitoring of targeted therapy in an individual patient. On the basis of the in vivo characterization of tumor biology determined by imaging, personalized medicine may become possible in cancer patients.

2.9 Conclusions

In this chapter we have outlined the role of imaging in the evaluation of tumor response to treatment, considering both the evolution of internationally accepted criteria for use in clinical trials and the potential of imaging modalities/techniques not included in these criteria. The limitations of standardized criteria were also discussed in the context of modern imaging techniques, which include a large spectrum of not only morphological but also functional methods for use either in the early phase or as final assessment. From this standpoint, we could expect a reduction in the time between the introduction of one formal system and the next: 20 years from WHO (1980) to RECIST 1.0 (2000), about 10 years to RECIST 1.1 (2009). How many years to the next RECIST (whether 1.2 or 2.0)? Yet, at least three important issues remain to be addressed.

Firstly, there is increasing use of new, targeted biological non-cytotoxic treatments that modify cell signaling pathways, thereby inhibiting cell growth. Note that these drugs do not kill the tumor cell: the aim is cancer control rather than elimination. This means that new therapies can determine SD, and not CR or PR. Tumor shrinkage should no longer be considered a major/unique index of response. In fact, the use of classical morphological/dimensional criteria in clinical trials may cause new drugs to be wrongly declared as ineffective.

This change in perspective is confirmed by the growing interest of oncologists in "the time that a cancer did not grow or metastasize further- that is, the length of time before progression occurred" [1]. This is the underlying reason why progression-free survival has become a popular end-point for clinical trials in oncology [54]. Thus SD, previously used to demonstrate therapy failure, is now used to demonstrate therapy success. This also means that we should consider a quantitative measure of response rather than a dichotomous subdivision between responders and non-responders. Moreover, especially when functional/metabolic imaging serves as the basis for an early prognostic index, what is the standard of reference? Which statistical methods? In order to evaluate the predictive ability of a test for future events, should we use methods for time-to-event/survival analysis (hazard and cumulative hazard functions, such as Cox regression, censoring, log-rank, etc.) or time-dependent receiver operating characteristic analysis [1]?

Imaging-based measurement of biological functions highlights the second remaining problem. In imaging for oncology, but also in all other imaging fields, a shift from qualitative to quantitative imaging is underway. As our reports become increasingly standardized they will include numbers, frequently obtained by means of dedicated software. Thus, it is unlikely that tumor response evaluation will be limited to 1D diameters. Obviously, quantitative methods, including the spectrum of indices described above and others now in development, will have to be standardized and verified in terms of reproducibility.

However, while standardized criteria have been proposed (and discussed) for clinical trials, what about clinical practice, outside the trials setting? The use of imaging as a surrogate endpoint in clinical practice requires the demonstration of a significant relationship between imaging results and clinical outcome. In the era of evidence-based medicine, prospective randomized clinical trials (RCTs) should be mandatory for this purpose. At the moment, large, well-designed prospective RCTs aimed at demonstrating an impact on patient outcome of imaging modalities in therapy monitoring are not available in the literature. We know that ethical, logistical, and financial concerns have to be addressed. But it is hard to accept that imaging modalities are used for selecting new anticancer treatments but lack of high-quality demonstrations such as RCTs to allow a better patient outcome in clinical practice. Cooperation between the pharmaceutical and the instrumentation industries is needed to support such trials, with funding sought from national and international agencies.

Third, can we translate standardized criteria into clinical practice in oncologic imaging? It is not easy to transfer the rigid rules designed for trials into a practice in which, at the very least, the intervals between one time point and the next may differ from those defined in the guidelines. However, efforts in this direction should be made, while emphasizing simplification, especially a reduction in the number of target lesions, as is the case in RECIST 1.1.

As recently stated by Sullivan and Gatsonis [1], "the pace of investigation and changes in our understanding of the molecular biology of cancer demand improved measure of response." We cannot ignore the advancements in hybrid imaging achieved with the introduction of hybrid PET/MRI systems. The combination of a functional (PET) with a morphological and functional modality (MRI) result in intrinsically co-registered *fusion* imaging [55, 56]. As this modality gains acceptance, will we still be able to judge tumor response to treatment mainly in terms of 1D diameters?

References

1. Sullivan DC, Gatsonis C (2011) Response to treatment series: part 1 and introduction, measuring tumor response challenges in the era of molecular medicine. AJR Am J Roentgenol 197:15-17
2. Sardanelli F, Di Leo G (2009) Biostatistics for Radiologists. Springer-Verlag, Milan, pp 142-144, 128-129
3. World Health Organization (1979) WHO handbook of reporting results of cancer treatment. World Health Organization, Geneva, Switzerland
4. Miller AB, Hoogstraten B, Staquet M, Winkler A (1981) Reporting results of cancer treatment. Cancer 47:207-214

5. Therasse P, Arbuck SG, Eisenhauer EA et al (2000) New guidelines to evaluate the response to treatment in solid tumors: European Organization for Research and Treatment of Cancer, National Cancer Institute of the United States, National Cancer Institute of Canada. J Natl Cancer Inst 92:205-216

6. Eisenhauer EA, Therasse P, Bogaerts J et al (2009) New response evaluation criteria in solid tumours: revised RECIST guideline (version 1.1). Eur J Cancer 45:228-247

7. Sardanelli F (2012) Evidence-based radiology and its relation to quality. In: Abujudeh HH, Bruno MA (eds) Quality and safety in radiology. Oxford University Press, New York, Chapter 27

8. Sardanelli F, Hunink MG, Gilbert FJ et al (2010) Evidence-based radiology: why and how? Eur Radiol 20:1-15

9. Wahl RL, Jacene H, Kasamon Y, Lodge MA (2009) From RECIST to PERCIST: Evolving Considerations for PET response criteria in solid tumors. J Nucl Med 50 Suppl 1:122S-150S

10. Nishino M, Jackman DM, Hatabu H et al (2010) New Response Evaluation Criteria in Solid Tumors (RECIST) guidelines for advanced non-small cell lung cancer: comparison with original RECIST and impact on assessment of tumor response to targeted therapy. AJR Am J Roentgenol 195:W221-228

11. Bruix J, Sherman M, Llovet JM et al; EASL Panel of Experts on HCC (2001) Clinical management of hepatocellular carcinoma: conclusions of the Barcelona-2000 EASL conference - European Association for the Study of the Liver. J Hepatol 35:421-430

12. Choi H, Charnsangavej C, de Castro Faria S et al (2004) CT evaluation of the response of gastrointestinal stromal tumors after imatinib mesylate treatment: a quantitative analysis correlated with FDG PET findings. AJR Am J Roentgenol 183:1619-1628

13. Lencioni R, Llovet JM (2010) Modified RECIST (mRECIST) assessment for hepatocellular carcinoma. Semin Liver Dis 30:52-60

14. Kudo M, Kubo S, Takayasu K et al; Liver Cancer Study Group of Japan (2010) Response Evaluation Criteria in Cancer of the Liver (RECICL) proposed by the Liver Cancer Study Group of Japan (2009 Revised Version). Hepatol Res 40:686-692

15. Apfaltrer P, Meyer M, Meier C et al (2012) Contrast-enhanced dual-energy CT of gastrointestinal stromal tumors: Is Iodine-related attenuation a potential indicator of tumor response? Invest Radiol 47:65-70

16. Nishino M, Jagannathan JP, Ramaiya NH, Van den Abbeele AD (2010) Revised RECIST guideline version 1.1: What oncologists want to know and what radiologists need to know. AJR Am J Roentgenol 195:281-289

17. Crabb SJ, Patsios D, Sauerbrei E et al (2009) Tumor cavitation: impact on objective response evaluation in trials of angiogenesis inhibitors in nonsmall-cell lung cancer. J Clin Oncol 27:404-410

18. Kambadakone AR, Sahani DV (2009) Body perfusion CT: technique, clinical applications, and advances. Radiol Clin North Am 47:161-178

19. Wu GY, Ghimire P (2009) Perfusion computed tomography in colorectal cancer: protocols, clinical applications and emerging trends. World J Gastroenterol 15:3228-3231

20. Okada M, Kim T, Murakami T (2011) Hepatocellular nodules in liver cirrhosis: state of the art CT evaluation (perfusion CT/volume helical shuttle scan/dual-energy CT, etc.). Abdom Imaging 36:273-281

21. Parodi RC, Sardanelli F, Renzetti P et al (2002) Growing Region Segmentation Software (GRES) for quantitative magnetic resonance imaging of multiple sclerosis: intra- and inter-observer agreement variability: a comparison with manual contouring method. Eur Radiol 12:866-871

22. Parodi RC, Levrero F, Sormani MP et al (2008) Supervised automatic procedure to identify new lesions in brain MR longitudinal studies of patients with multiple sclerosis. Radiol Med 113:300-306

23. Monsky WL, Kim I, Loh S et al (2010) Semiautomated segmentation for volumetric analysis of intratumoral ethiodol uptake and subsequent tumor necrosis after chemoembolization. AJR Am J Roentgenol 195:1220-1230

24. Vignati A, Giannini V, De Luca M et al (2011) Performance of a fully automatic lesion detection system for breast DCE-MRI. J Magn Reson Imaging 34:1341-1351
25. Kuhl CK (2007) Current status of breast MR imaging. I. Choice of technique, image interpretation, diagnostic accuracy, and transfer to clinical practice. Radiology 244:672–691
26. Tofts PS, Brix G, Buckley DL (1999) Estimating kinetic parameters from dynamic contrast-enhanced T(1)-weighted MRI of a diffusable tracer: standardized quantities and symbols. J Magn Reson Imaging 10:223-232
27. Sardanelli F, Serafin Z, Stoker J (2012) Evidence-based radiology 2001-2010: The authorship. Abstract, ECR 2012
28. Woodhams R, Kakita S, Hata H et al (2010) Identification of residual breast carcinoma following neoadjuvant chemotherapy: diffusion-weighted imaging – comparison with contrast-enhanced MR imaging and pathologic findings. Radiology 254:357-366
29. Afaq A, Andreou A, Koh DM (2010) Diffusion-weighted magnetic resonance imaging for tumour response assessment: why, when and how? Cancer Imaging 10 Spec no A:S179-88
30. Thoeny HC, Ross BD (2010) Predicting and monitoring cancer treatment response with diffusion-weighted MRI. J Magn Reson Imaging 32:2-16
31. Lambregts DM, Maas M, Cappendijk VC et al (2011) Whole-body diffusion-weighted magnetic resonance imaging: current evidence in oncology and potential role in colorectal cancer staging. Eur J Cancer 47:2107-2116
32. Glunde K, Jiang L, Moestue SA, Gribbestad IS (2011) MRS and MRSI guidance in molecular medicine: targeting and monitoring of choline and glucose metabolism in cancer. NMR Biomed 24:673-690
33. King AD, Yeung DK, Yu KH et al (2010) Pretreatment and early intratreatment prediction of clinicopathologic response of head and neck cancer to chemoradiotherapy using 1H-MRS. J Magn Reson Imaging 32:199-203
34. Baek HM, Chen JH, Nalcioglu O, Su MY (2008) Proton MR spectroscopy for monitoring early treatment response of breast cancer to neo-adjuvant chemotherapy. Ann Oncol 19:1022-1024
35. Podo F, Sardanelli F, Iorio E et al (2007) Abnormal choline ohospholipid metabolism in breast and ovary cancer: Molecular bases for noninvasive imaging approaches. Curr Med Imaging Reviews 3:123-137
36. Sardanelli F, Fausto A, Di Leo G et al (2009) In vivo proton MR spectroscopy of the breast using the total choline peak integral as a marker of malignancy. AJR Am J Roentgenol 192:1608-1617
37. Esseridou A, Di Leo G, Sconfienza LM et al (2011) In vivo detection of choline in ovarian tumors using 3D magnetic resonance spectroscopy. Invest Radiol 46:377-382
38. Marcus Marcus CD, Ladam-Marcus V, Cucu C et al (2009). Imaging techniques to evaluate the response to treatment in oncology: current standards and perspectives. Crit Rev Oncol Hematol 72:217-238
39. Kim CK, Choi D, Lim HK et al (2005) Therapeutic response assessment of percutaneous radiofrequency ablation for hepatocellular carcinoma: utility of contrast-enhanced agent detection imaging. Eur J Radiol 56:66-73
40. Lamuraglia M, Escudier B, Chami L et al (2006) To predict progression-free survival and overall survival in metastatic renal cancer treated with sorafenib: pilot study using dynamic contrast-enhanced Doppler ultrasound. Eur J Cancer 42:2472-2479
41. Lassau N, Koscielny S, Chami L et al (2011) Advanced hepatocellular carcinoma: early evaluation of response to bevacizumab therapy at dynamic contrast-enhanced US with quantification—preliminary results. Radiology 258:291-300
42. Williams R, Hudson JM, Lloyd BA et al (2011) Dynamic microbubble contrast-enhanced US to measure tumor response to targeted therapy: a proposed clinical protocol with results from renal cell carcinoma patients receiving antiangiogenic therapy. Radiology 260:581-590
43. Ell PJ (2006) The contribution of PET/CT to improved patient management. Br J Radiol 79:32-36

44. Brown RS, Wahl RL (1993) Overexpression of Glut-1 glucose transporter in human breast cancer. An immunohistochemical study. Cancer 72:2979-2985

45. Higashi K, Clavo AC, Wahl RL (1993) Does FDG uptake measure proliferative activity of human cancer cells? In vitro comparison with DNA flow cytometry and tritiated thymidine uptake. J Nucl Med 34:414-419

46. Brucher BL, Weber W, Bauer M et al (2001) Neoadjuvant therapy of esophageal squamous cell carcinoma: response evaluation by positron emission tomography. Ann Surg 233:300-309

47. Bos R, van Der Hoeven JJ, van Der Wall E et al (2002) Biologic correlates of (18)fluo-rodeoxyglucose uptake in human breast cancer measured by positron emission tomography. J Clin Oncol 20:379-387

48. Blodgett TM, Ryan A (2009) Pitfalls and limitations. In: Blodgett TM (ed) Specialty imaging. PET/CT oncologic imaging with correlative diagnostic CT. Amirsys, Salt Lake City

49. Herrmann K, Krause BJ, Bundschuh RA et al (2009) Monitoring response to therapeutic interventions in patients with cancer. Semin Nucl Med 39:210-232

50. Vriens D, Visser EP, de Geus-Oei LF, Oyen WJ (2010) Methodological considerations in quantification of oncological FDG PET studies. Eur J Nucl Med Mol Imaging 37:1408-1425

51. Zasadny KR, Wahl RL (1993) Standardized uptake values of normal tissues at PET with 2-[fluorine-18]-fluoro-2-deoxy-d-glucose: variations with body weight and a method for correction. Radiology 189:847-850

52. Ford EC, Kinahan PE, Hanlon L et al (2006) Tumor delineation using PET in head and neck cancers: threshold contouring and lesion volumes. Med Phys 33:4280-4288

53. Boellaard R, O'Doherty MJ, Weber WA et al (2010). FDG PET and PET/CT: EANM procedure guidelines for tumour PET imaging: version 1.0. Eur J Nucl Med Mol Imaging 37:181-200

54. Lebwohl D, Kay A, Berg W et al (2009) Progression-free survival: gaining on overall survival as a gold standard and accelerating drug development. Cancer J 15:386-394

55. Sullivan DC, Gatsonis C (2011) Response to treatment series: part 1 and introduction, measuring tumor response-challenges in the era of molecular medicine. AJR Am J Roentgenol 197:15-17

56. Wolf W (2011) The unique potential for noninvasive imaging in modernizing drug development and in transforming therapeutics: PET/MRI/MRS. Pharm Res 28:490-493

57. Sauter AW, Wehrl HF, Kolb A, Judenhofer MS, Pichler BJ (2010) Combined PET/MRI: one step further in multimodality imaging. Trends Mol Med 16:508-515

Part II

RECIST and Beyond: Assessing the Response to Treatment in Metastatic Disease

Gastrointestinal Stromal Tumors

3

Giovanni Grignani, Paola Boccone, Teresio Varetto
and Stefano Cirillo

3.1   Introduction

Gastrointestinal stromal tumor (GIST) is the most common mesenchymal tumor of the gastrointestinal tract. According to tumor size, GIST incidence varies from a highly prevalent tumor the "micro-GIST," which is < 2 cm wide [1] and is estimated to occur in up to 22% of the general population, to a rare disease characterized by a tumor > 2 cm and with an annual incidence of about 15/1,000,000 [2]. While the clinical relevance of microGIST is still under evaluation, at this point it is considered to be minimal. GISTs may develop from the esophagus to the rectum and are most common in the stomach (60–70% of the cases) followed by the small intestine (30%), and lastly by the rectum (< 10%) [3]. Although no GIST > 2 cm can be considered benign, the risk of local relapse and metastasis varies according to tumor size and site of origin, and the number of mitoses evaluated on 50 microscopic high-power fields. This risk stratification proposed by Miettinen and Lasota [3] is widely used as a prognosticator after complete surgery, which is still the mainstay of therapy. However, despite complete surgical removal of the tumor, the 50% relapse rate is surprisingly consistent throughout different large series [4]. Relapse may occur locally but mostly involves the peritoneum and liver. Patients with relapse not amenable to surgery previously died within 12 months [5] due to the chemoresistance of GIST, in which the response rate to chemotherapy is < 5% [6].

However, after Hirota et al. [7] showed that GIST proliferation was caused by constitutive activation of the type III tyrosine kinase (TRK) receptor KIT in nearly all tumors and less often by the platelet-derived growth factor recep-

G. Grignani (✉)
Division of Medical Oncology, Institute for Cancer Research and Treatment (IRCC),
Candiolo (Turin), Italy

tor-α(PDGFR-α) [8], new approaches to the treatment of this rare disease were attempted. An extraordinarily successful treatment of a woman with widespread GIST with the KIT inhibitor imatinib was reported on the New England Journal of Medicine in 2001 [9]. Since the publication of this case report, imatinib has become the unquestionable model of targeted therapy with small-molecule inhibitors. Two extensive phase III studies showed that imatinib was active and effective in advanced GIST, sharply increasing both progression-free survival and overall survival [10, 11]. An earlier phase II study had shown that the heterogeneity of GISTs could be explained by the presence and the type of mutation of their oncogenes [12]. Thus, a spectrum of genetically different diseases is currently recognized, in which mutations in different oncogenes and different types of mutations nonetheless give rise to the same pathological entity [13]. In the imatinib era, this new classification of GISTs represents an extraordinary clinical tool in disease management. Indeed, the molecular information on which it is based confirms the importance of a multidisciplinary, patient-tailored therapeutic approach in order to achieve the best possible results according to the different presentations of this tumor. International guidelines [14, 15] classify GISTs as localized, locally advanced or metastatic. Based on disease extension and site of origin, the proposed clinical management may vary considerably.

3.2   Therapeutic Strategy

In localized GIST, surgery is still the first and most critical approach, as it must guarantee adequate margins and minimize the risk of tumor rupture (which may also occur spontaneously) given that tumor spilling implies a 95% risk of relapse [16]. The surgical feasibility of adequate margins and tumor rupture also guides clinical decision-making for patients with locally advanced GISTs. Moreover, since imatinib may shrink the tumor, patients initially treated with the drug may require less aggressive surgery, with the possibility of functional sparing (i.e., avoiding total gastrectomy or perineal-abdominal amputation). The safety and results of this neo-adjuvant approach have been published by different groups [17]. In metastatic disease, there is no role for surgery, or, at most, as an exploratory measure on an individualized basis. Nevertheless, in patients with metastatic GIST imatinib may sometimes shrink the tumor as well as the metastases to an extent that allows complete excision of all detectable disease. This possibilty has been explored by different groups and, once again, the results have been very similar [18-20].

It is therefore clear that imatinib mesylate is the cornerstone of the clinical strategy in patients with GIST. The success of this drug is due to the higher incidence in GIST of mutations in exons 9 and 11 of KIT, which predicts the achievement of stable disease in nearly 85% of the patients. Indeed, the underlying genotype is of the greatest relevance in predicting outcome. Thus, a wild-type or resistant genotype (e.g., PDGFR-α exon-18 D842V) sharply reduces or abrogates any role for the currently available targeted therapies [21]. In general, four different therapeutic scenarios can be described: the adjuvant setting, the neo-adjuvant setting, advanced disease, and beyond multikinase inhibitor failure.

3.2.1 Adjuvant Therapy

Patients receiving 400 mg of imatinib for 1 year have prolonged recurrence-free survival after complete surgery of a tumor of almost any size [22]. Unplanned analyses have shown that there is no advantage for tumors bearing exon-9 mutation and for wild-type GIST, whereas almost all other subtypes achieve an advantage by medical therapy after surgery. At the 2011 ASCO meeting, Joensuu [23] presented the results obtained in GIST patients administered imatinib at the same dose for 3 years, concluding that relapse-free and overall survival were prolonged in patients with high-risk and very high-risk GISTs.

3.2.2 Neo-adjuvant Therapy

Soon after the publication of the B2222 data [14], it became clear that patients with either large or critically located (e.g., rectum) GIST could benefit from tumor shrinkage and thus from imatinib therapy. In an attempt to improve the quality of surgery and to reduce related morbidity, candidates for surgery were pre-operatively treated with imatinib. However, 10 years later, a formal proof for the success of this strategy is still lacking. Nonetheless, based on small mono-institutional series, it remains a commonly accepted integrated approach to minimize surgical damage or inadequate results [14].

3.2.3 Advanced Disease

In these patients, tumor genotype guides medical therapy. Thus, tumors with an exon 11 mutation are best treated with a daily dose of 400 mg of imatinib whereas those with an exon 9 mutation require 800 mg daily [24]. In GISTs arising from a mutated PDGFR-α, the standard dose is 400 mg daily, but there is a well-known mutation affecting exon-18 (D842V) that is refractory to imatinib therapy. Wild-type GISTs have a lower sensitivity to imatinib therapy, but there is no indication supporting an increase in the imatinib dose. However, the problem remains that secondary imatinib resistance develops in less than 24 months in 50% of the patients. Consequently, there is a large consensus to double the dose of imatinib, if initiated at 400 mg [25], and, in case of failure, to start therapy with the TRK inhibitor sunitinib malate 50 mg daily for 4 weeks on and 2 weeks off or at a dose of 37.5 mg on a continuous daily base [26, 27].

3.2.4   Beyond Multikinase Inhibitor Failure

Patients whose disease does not respond to sunitinib are offered as-yet experimental third-line therapies based on the multikinase inhibitors sorafenib, regorafenib, and dasatinib [28, 29]. None of these drugs is approved for clinical use. Recently, a phase III trial demonstrated a statistically significant advantage of masatinib over sunitinib as a third-line therapy. Since these data are preliminary and not yet available in the literature, they should be interpreted with caution. Currently, the preferred approach in patients with progression after sunitinib and/or other inhibitors is to re-challenge the GISTs with the highest tolerated dose of imatinib. Although not evidence-based, this treatment option may delay progression, by the action of the drug on still sensitive neoplastic clones.

3.3   The Issue of Targeted Therapy Response Evaluation

In this complex and multidisciplinary approach, it is clear that the imaging evaluation of GIST is of utmost importance. Imaging along with the pathology report guides clinical decision-making and after staging it defines the first-line therapy. Thereafter, it allows monitoring of the response guiding the integration of medical and surgical therapies. This is a crucial point in all GISTs, in light of the report [9] that despite the unprecedented activity of imatinib it did not necessarily cause tumor shrinkage, as often observed after traditional forms of chemotherapy. Consequently, dimensional criteria such as RECIST, while certainly useful and reproducible, may be only belatedly applicable since changes in tumor dimension may first occur later in the course of treatment. Therefore, dimension per se might not help in the early identification of responders. This limitation is also relevant when therapy is not effective. TRK inhibitors are expensive and toxic and they should be discontinued in patients with resistant disease, which might be better treated with other drugs. Clearly, the ability to identify responsive patients is a clinical issue and not only an academic one. Any effort to improve our understanding of TRK activity is a step forward in the better clinical use of these innovative therapies.

Thus, rather than tumor shrinkage, pathological and functional/molecular response are probably better tools to objectively identify and measure imatinib activity earlier and more accurately. In fact, as reported by Mankoff et al. in 2007 [30], tumor shrinkage is only the final step in a complex cascade of cellular and subcellular changes after imatinib treatment. Molecular imaging could play an important role in the evaluation of the cellular changes occurring in the early stages of treatment. For example, it could detect decreases in cell proliferation, increases in cell death, and a decline in the number of viable tumor cells. This approach considers that while targeted therapies reduce GIST diameters, this might occur as late as months after the initiation of therapy. Accordingly, the evaluation of response based solely on dimensional criteria is not as accurate as in other oncological settings. In light of these conclusions, a need was recognized for imaging strategies that improve the readout of imatinib activity and thus for criteria to identify patients benefiting from treatment [31-35]. This effort has proven to be of great value not only in patients receiving imatinib therapy, but also in those treated with other kinase inhibitors [36]. Moreover, the success of these efforts extends beyond GIST to other types of tumors [37].

3.4   A CT Assessment of the Response to Treatment: The RECIST Criteria

Several imaging modalities are available to assess the response to therapy in patients with metastatic GIST. As discussed in Chap. 2, imaging can yield anatomical/topographical or functional/molecular information. In GIST, the most commonly used modality to follow these patients is CT, which allows assessment of both the side effects of targeted therapies and the response to treatment [38]. Both in the initial staging and during follow-up, CT should be performed following a bolus injection of iodine contrast material using a triphasic protocol. The arterial phase begins 35–40 s from the start of the injection, and the portal phase 70–75 s post-injection. Since the most common site of metastasization is the liver, where lesions are usually hypervascular, these tumors are best appreciated in arterial phase while often go undetected in portal phase (Fig. 3.1a).

In the last ten years, the response to treatment of GISTs has been evaluated, as for other tumors, using the RECIST criteria [39]. However, as noted above, there are several pitfalls in the assessment of GIST by means of unidimensional criteria, since imatinib often induces cystic changes due to myxoid degeneration. At CT, changes in lesion density and size, with tumor liquefaction, may be observed. Here, the potential pitfalls reflect the fact that at this stage there may be an increase in lesion size and an apparent increase in lesion number. Occasionally, hepatic metastases that were difficult to visualize on pre-treatment CT can be seen on follow-up CT scans as hypodense lesions, potentially misinterpreted as disease progression (Fig. 3.1). As previously reported for other cancers, it is important to underline that the inter-observer variability in the measurement of tumor size in patients receiving imatinib therapy is very high [40].

Compared to the other imaging techniques, CT plays a key role in evaluating treatment response as well as therapy-related adverse effects. CT can show the adverse effects of TRK inhibitors, which, in general are limited to minor ascites and pleural and pericardial effusion (Figs. 3.2, 3.3).

However, in < 5% of patients with bulky tumors, there may be severe intratumoral bleeding requiring surgical treatment (Fig. 3.4). Other important complications are massive necrosis with perforation or abscess formation [38].

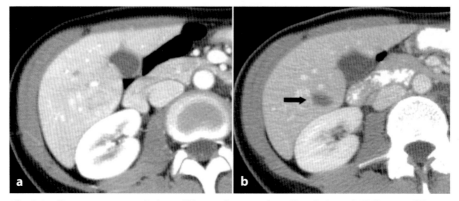

Fig. 3.1 a Pre-treatment portal phase CT scan does not show liver lesions. **b** Follow-up CT, performed after therapy with imatinib, shows a 2 cm hypodense lesion in the medial aspect of segment 6 (*arrow*). In GIST, the appearance of new liver lesions is not always a sign of disease progression

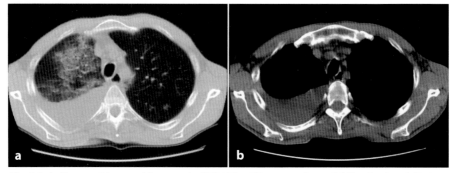

Fig. 3.2 A 49-year-old man with a gastric GIST. The CT scan performed following imatinib therapy shows (**a**) consolidation in the upper right lobe and (**b**) right-sided pleural effusion

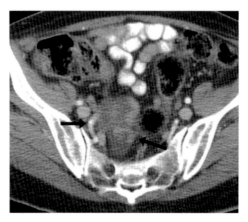

Fig. 3.3 A 67-year-old male with gastric GIST: CT after imatinib therapy shows the appearance of ascites, a collateral effect of therapy

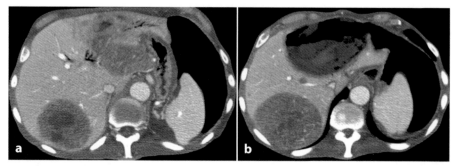

Fig. 3.4 A 71-year-old man with gastric GIST and several large hepatic metastases. **a** Following imatinib therapy, CT shows a pneumoperitoneum due to intestinal perforation. **b** A second, more caudal CT scan shows a large necrotic liver metastasis connecting to the peritoneal cavity

3.5 New Approaches in CT Monitoring of the Response to Targeted Therapies

Several reports have shown that RECIST criteria may underestimate the extent of response to new targeted therapies [33, 38, 41-44]. GIST lesions have been shown to initially increase in size following imatinib therapy, even in cases of a favorable outcome, due to intratumoral necrosis or bleeding (Fig. 3.5) [38]. In a landmark contribution, Choi et al. [33] compared unidimensional RECIST criteria, tumor CT attenuation coefficient, and ^{18}F-FDG PET to clinical endpoints. No significant difference was observed in the long-term prognosis of good vs. poor responders, when the RECIST criteria were used. Conversely, when tumor response was evaluated on the basis of a combination of tumor

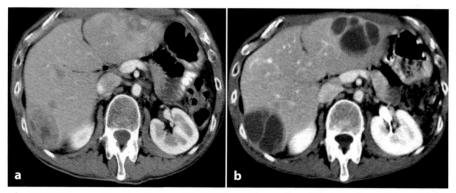

Fig. 3.5 A 56-year-old male with a gastric GIST. **a** After the identification of hepatic metastases, the patient was started on imatinib at a daily dose of 400 mg. **b** After 2 months of therapy, the CT image showed a significant increase in the size of two metastases but a concomitant density reduction, indicating that treatment may have been effective

Table 3.1 Choi CT criteria to assess response to imatinib treatment (modified from [33])

Type of response	CHOI Criteria (after 2 months of therapy)
Complete response	Disappearance of all lesions, no new lesion
PR	A decrease in size of ≥ 10% or a decrease in tumor density (HU) ≥ 15% on CT, no new lesions, no obvious progression of non-measurable disease
SD	Does not meet the criteria for complete response, partial response or progressive disease, no symptomatic deterioration attributed to tumor progression
Progressive disease	An increase in tumor size of ≥ 10% and does not meet criteria of partial response by tumor density (HU) on CT, new lesions, new intratumoral nodules or an increase in the size of the existing intratumoral nodules

PR, partial response; *SD,* stable disease.

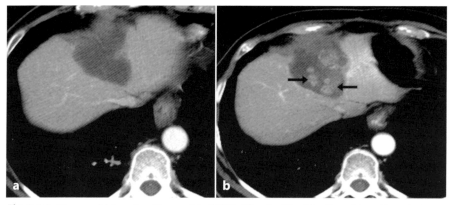

Fig. 3.6 A 64-year-old female with a gastric GIST. After the identification of hepatic metastases, the patient was started on 400 mg of imatinib, administered daily. The CT scan after 2 months of therapy (**a**) and after 12 months of therapy (**b**). The appearance of enhanced nodules (*arrows*) within a responsive tumoral lesion over time is a sign of disease progression

size and tumor density, a significant difference in the long-term prognosis of good vs. poor responders was observed. In particular a reduction in tumor size > 10% and a decrease in the attenuation coefficient of > 15% in the 2 months after treatment had a sensitivity of 97% (vs. 52% for the RECIST criteria) and a specificity of 100% in detecting responders. On the basis of these data, Choi et al. [33] suggested new, modified CT response evaluation criteria based not only on 1D measurements but also on changes in CT density (Table 3.1).

According to the Choi criteria, the appearance of new enhanced nodules within the tumor, an increase in the solid part of the tumor, and an increase in tumor vascularization are all signs of disease progression (Fig. 3.6) [33].

In summary, parameters such as tumor density, size, vascularization, and intratumoral nodules allow the radiologist to correctly assess treatment response [45]. However, the prognostic value of the Choi criteria have yet to be determined. In a recent study, Dudeck et al. [46] demonstrated that patients classified as having a stable disease according to RECIST criteria had a similar progression-free survival and overall survival as patients classified as partial responders or with stable disease according to the Choi criteria. Other limitations of these criteria are their inappropriateness in the evaluation of secondary relapses [47] and the potential effects on density values due to the presence of intratumoral hemorrhage.

3.6 Therapy Response Evaluation with ^{18}F-FDG PET/CT

In the last few years several studies have compared the value of PET and CT in detecting tumor response to therapy in patients with GIST. In 2004, Antoch et al. [48] used the WHO, RECIST and EORTC criteria to evaluate response in 20 patients with GIST who underwent ^{18}F-FDG PET/CT before and 1, 3, and 6 months after the start of imatinib therapy. The combination of PET and CT images showed the highest accuracy. Indeed, the number of lesions detected by CT and PET alone and by fused PET/CT at baseline was 135, 249, and 282, respectively. PET/CT correctly characterized tumor response in 95% of patients at 1 month and in 100% after 3 and 6 months; PET correctly evaluated therapy response in 85% of patients at 1 month and in 100% at 3 and 6 months; finally, CT accurately diagnosed tumor response only in 44% of the patients at 1 month, in 60% at 3 months, and in 57% at 6 months. In the same year, Choi et al. [49] correlated changes in tumor density on CT with changes in glucose metabolism on ^{18}F-FDG PET. In responders, they showed the occurrence of a significant decrease in both tumor density and SUV_{max}. Although no statistically significant association was found between these two parameters, 70% of the patients with tumors that showed response to ^{18}F-FDG PET demonstrated at least a partial response using the tumor density criteria, while 75% of the patients were classified as having stable disease according to the RECIST criteria. Gayed et al. [50] compared PET with CT in 49 patients 2 months after completion of imatinib therapy. PET was shown to predict the response to therapy earlier than CT in 22.5% of patients. Lastly, Holdsworth et al. [51] studied 63 patients with GIST who underwent PET and CT imaging studies after 1 month of treatment. In this patient group, the time to treatment failure was best predicted by a SUV_{max} threshold of 3.4 at 1 month ($p = 0.0001$) and a reduction in the SUV_{max} of 40% ($p = 0.0002$) [51]. Their results suggested that conventional objective response criteria are not generally applicable to prognosis in therapies involving the new molecularly targeted agents.

3.6.1 Early Response Assessment and Prediction of Response

Experimental data have shown that the exposure of GIST cells to imatinib results in a rapid decline of GLUT-2 receptor recruitment to the cell membrane; GLUT-2 has been identified as the principal glucose transporter in GIST cells

[52]. Using a small-animal model, Cullinane et al. [53] were able to demonstrate that FDG uptake into tumors expressing the c-KIT V560G mutation was significantly reduced as early as 4 h after the beginning of imatinib treatment. Clinically, some studies showed that a GIST response to imatinib is associated with a rapid reduction in FDG uptake, preceding changes in conventional response criteria by several weeks [50]. In the clinical scenario, ^{18}F-FDG PET response could be appreciated as early as day 8 after the initiation of imatinib (Fig. 3.7); PET responders had a significantly longer progression-free survival at one year than non-responders (92% *vs*. 12% respectively) [54].

In 2004, Goerres et al. [55] observed that patients responding to treatment, as measured by normalization of FDG-avid areas, had a better clinical outcome than patients in whom FDG uptake persisted. Indeed, in their study the median survival of patients with an ^{18}F-FDG PET response was 100% at 2 years compared to 49% in the group with residual tumor uptake. The authors also compared the prognostic significance of PET and contrast-enhanced CT in 28 patients, concluding that a single post-treatment PET scan, but not a single post-treatment contrast-enhanced CT scan, can provide prognostic information on overall survival and on time to progression. Indeed, the first follow-up CT was considered normal in only two of 28 patients. The measurement of changes between pre-treatment PET and the first follow-up PET scan and between pre-treatment CT and the first follow-up CT scan showed a significant

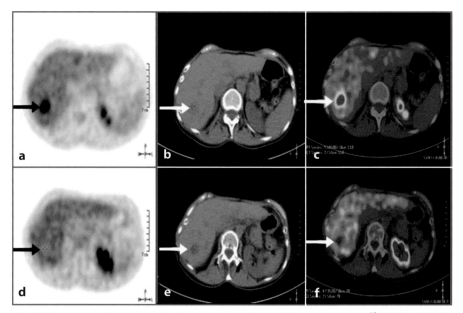

Fig. 3.7 Sixty-year-old woman with liver metastases from GIST. **a** At baseline ^{18}F-FDG PET/CT shows focal uptake in segment 6. **b** Non-contrast CT shows a hypodense lesion in the same liver segment. **c** Correlation between PET and CT images is confirmed by the fusion image. **d-f** After one week of 400 imatinib PET shows complete metabolic response

role only for PET imaging in predicting the overall survival of responders (PET changes: log-rank test $p = 0.009$; CT changes: log-rank test $p = 0.706$). More recently, Prior et al. [36] found that a PET scan performed 4 weeks after initiating treatment with sunitinib after imatinib failure is useful for the early assessment of treatment response and for the prediction of clinical outcome in GIST patients. In their study, progression-free survival correlated with early ^{18}F-FDG PET metabolic response; when a single ^{18}F-FDG PET was considered after 4 weeks of sunitinib, median progression-free survival was 29 weeks for SUVs < 8 g/mL vs. 4 weeks for SUVs ≥ 8 g/mL ($p < 0.0001$) [36].

3.6.2   Caveats in ^{18}F-FDG PET/CT Response Assessment

On PET/CT, response is characterized by a decrease in FDG uptake, with the measurement of SUV used to quantify the decrease. However it is important to underline that a positive baseline PET/CT examination is a prerequisite in therapy evaluation, as not all GIST lesions display appreciable glucose uptake. Furthermore, small lesions can occasionally be difficult to detect within bowel folds, in the pelvis, or in the omentum. SUV measurements are subject to variability related to the determination of a region of interest (ROI) by the test interpreter. A strong standardization of acquisitions and interpretation procedures along with the assessment of variability across readers should be conducted before intitiating ^{18}F-FDG PET response assessments.

3.7   Emerging Imaging Techniques in the Assessment of Response to Treatment in Patients with GIST

The role of MRI in assessing early treatment response has been recently evaluated. Tang et al. [56] investigated the apparent diffusion coefficient (ADC, see Chapter 2) as a predictor of early response in patients with GIST. The authors observed a significant increase in ADC values in responding lesions vs. a very modest increase in the poor-response group (44.8% vs. 1.5% at week 1), thus concluding that a marked increase in the ADC values 1 week after the beginning of imatinib therapy is associated with a good response. Technical advances now allow whole-body DW-MRI to be performed on a routine basis (Fig. 3.8). In the future, this new technique will likely play a key role in diseases staging and in the evaluation of treatment response [57].

A pilot study recently evaluated CT perfusion patterns in GIST lesions in patients undergoing therapy with sunitinib and imatinib [58]. With respect to extrahepatic and hepatic lesions, perfusion was significantly lower in good responders than in poor responders. The authors concluded that CT perfusion could in the future be adopted as a biomarker for treatment response.

Dual-energy CT allows the evaluation of iodine-related attenuation (IRA), which can be considered as a surrogate of perfusion and vascularization; in

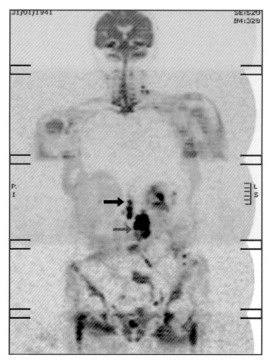

Fig. 3.8 A 58-year-old man with a GIST in the small intestine. Whole-body DW-MRI shows the primary tumor as well as the peritoneal metastases (*gray* and *black arrows*, respectively)

fact, the amount of iodinated contrast medium in a tissue depends on the degree of vascularization. In a recent study, Apfaltrer et al. [59] demonstrated a good correlation between IRA and the Choi criteria: IRA appeared to be a more robust parameter of response than density because it is not influenced by intratumoral hemorrhage.

3.8   Imaging Assessment Proposal

Based on the specific contribution that each imaging technique gives to the assessment of GIST in the era of targeted therapy we propose the following guidelines.

Base line evaluation. In patients with advanced disease, the integration of CT and PET/CT certainly yields the highest amount of information regarding both the true extension of the disease and the interpretation of odd features of response, e.g. cystic transformation in pre-existing necrotic tissue. Moreover, ^{18}F-FDG PET/CT could allow early prediction of response to treatment.

Patients that are borderline for surgery, because of tumor in critical sites, (e.g. the rectum) or due to tumor size, may benefit the most from baseline assessment.

Ongoing therapy evaluation. In general, CT is a suitable instrument to confirm and monitor the benefit of ongoing therapy. Radiologists should look for any density changes and carefully evaluate the peritoneum, where the detection of new metastases is often more difficult. ^{18}F-FDG PET is more sensitive in detecting early progression after response. However, it is not yet demonstrated that this affects prognosis. We suggest that, whenever residual surgery is considered, ^{18}F-FDG PET be added to patient evaluation in order to increase the likelihood of detecting formerly unrecognized sites of disease.

Second/further line therapy evaluation. CT is the first level test to monitor patients with GIST. Given the lower therapeutic index of second-line therapies, it is clinically important to ascertain the degree of tumor control achieved by the administered drug. ^{18}F-FDG PET detects sunitinib activity earlier than CT, but early identification of response has not been proven to affect patient outcome.

3.9   Conclusions

The advent of targeted therapies has greatly altered the horizon of tumor therapy, from cellular destruction to cellular silencing. This innovation requires further improvement in our ability to detect intratumoral events so as to identify the patients who will genuinely benefit from these innovative but expensive therapies. The integration of CT, MRI, and PET/CT seems the most promising approach to more correctly stage and evaluate the response to imatinib and other multikinase inhibitors in patients with GIST.

Clinical Case

A 78-year-old female presented with abdominal discomfort. On ultrasound, a 20-cm-wide mass was visible in the mid-left abdominal quadrant in proximity to the pancreas and stomach, which were considered the two most likely site of origin. The neoplasm surrounded the upper mesenteric artery. An ultrasound-guided core biopsy was performed and histopathology confirmed a CD117-positive GIST with 15 mitoses per 50 high-power fields. A *KIT* exon 11 mutation was also detected. Staging was then completed with an abdominal CT scan and ^{18}F-FDG PET (Fig. 3.9).

Imatinib at a dose of 400 mg/day was started. After 1 week of treatment, the patient complained of abdominal pain and fluid retention, with a sharp body weight increase (+ 3 kg). An abdominal ultrasound did not show significant changes compared to the baseline study except for the presence of ascites, mostly in the pelvis. Imatinib was continued and nimesulide (200 mg daily) and furosemide (25 mg daily) were added, achieving pain and fluid-retention control. Therapy was then uneventfully continued. After 2 months, a CT scan showed a dimensional reduction (wider axis reduced from 20 to 15 cm), a sharp density reduction, and the appearance of hypodense hepatic metastases (Fig. 3.10). The radiologic features of these apparently new lesions raised the suspicion of a progressing disease despite the partial response of the primary tumor. However, this is a typical picture of response to targeted therapy in GIST, in which any tumoral lesion needs to be interpreted bearing in mind that isodense lesions may become readily detectable after therapy because of intense vascular collapse due to imatinib. Therefore, any apparently new lesion has to be, retrospectively, thoroughly searched and interpreted in

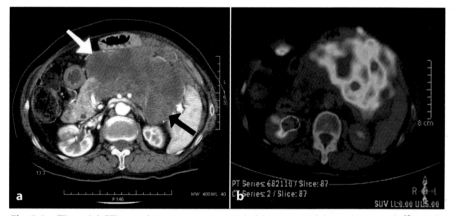

Fig. 3.9 a The axial CT scan shows an enormous primitive tumor of the peritoneum. **b** ^{18}F-FDG PET highlights the high metabolic activity of the lesion

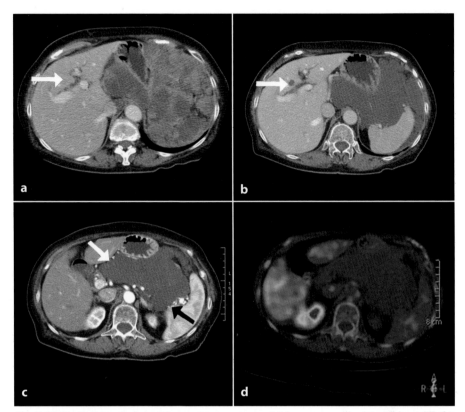

Fig. 3.10 An isodense lesion at the pre-treatment scan (**a**) became readily detectable at CT (**b**) after therapy, because of the intense vascular collapse mediated by imatinib. **c** A sharp decrease in the tumor density is observed also within the primitive lesion. **d** In the latter, there is no residual metabolic activity at ^{18}F-FDG PET

light of its radiological features, especially the density change. The patient remained on the same dose of imatinib for another 21 months, when a CT scan control showed a further shrinkage of the hypodense tumor (wider axis 12.5 cm) and the appearance of a new hyperdense nodule (Fig. 3.11a). The suspicion of localized disease progression was confirmed by a ^{18}F-FDG PET. Figure 3.11b shows a clear hot-spot within the large mass confirming the suspicion of disease progression. The radiological picture of a "nodule within a nodule" is a well-recognized sign of progression. Therefore, per se further ^{18}F-FDG PET confirmation is not required. In this context, PET may be used with a dual purpose: (1) to precociously identify progressive disease after a change in therapy; (2) in the case of local therapy aimed at controlling focal progression, to verify limited progression. In this patient, who at the time was 78 years old, ^{18}F-FDG PET was performed in order to quickly determine the potential ben-

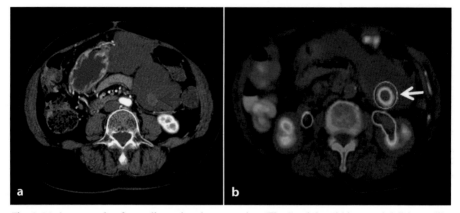

Fig. 3.11 An example of non-dimensional progression. The "nodule within a nodule" is readily appreciated both at CT (*red arrow*) (**a**) and ¹⁸F-FDG PET (*white arrow*) (**b**)

efit/failure of an increased dose of imatinib, as a daily dose of 800 mg can be difficult to maintain in the elderly due to anemia, fluid retention, and fatigue. The certainty of benefit can increase patient compliance as can tailoring the dose to the patient.

The imatinib dose was increased to 800 mg/day but had to be discontinued after 4 weeks due to fluid retention (increased body weight of 3.5 kg). Diuretics were started and after 5 days the patient was again administered imatinib, at a dose of 300 mg twice daily, which thereafter was maintained. After 6 weeks, the patient was re-evaluated by CT and ¹⁸F-FDG PET, which showed a complete response to the increased dose (Fig. 3.12). Unfortunately, a new metastasis had rapidly grown next to the abdominal wall. At the last follow-up, the patient, now on sunitinib 37.5 mg daily, had no evidences of further disease progression.

This case report demonstrates the different aspects of TRK inhibitor therapy. First, accurate initial imaging is a key aspect of disease management in later stages. Second, dimensional criteria are only one step in the radiological evaluation of the response to TKIs. Third, ¹⁸F-FDG PET may help in the interpretation of a mixed response or in case of focal progression, contributing to the clinical decision-making required by these challenging situations. Fourth, proactive adverse event management may substantially increase patient adherence to prescribed doses, which is crucial to achieving lasting disease control; an adjusted dose might allow frail patients, e.g. the elderly, to continue treatment for years. Finally, second-line treatment should be offered to elderly patients regardless of their co-morbidities tailoring the dosage to each single patient and to the side effects observed.

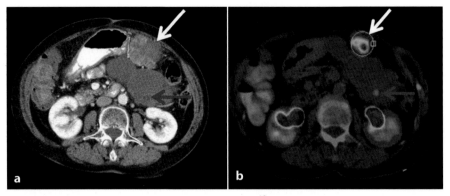

Fig. 3.12 After 6 weeks, both arterial phase CT (**a**) and ^{18}F-FDG PET (**b**) show a response at the previous site of disease (*red arrows*). However, a new lesion appeared in the anterior aspect of the peritoneal cavity (*white arrows*)

References

1. Agaimy A, Wünsch PH, Hofstaedter F et al (2007) Minute gastric sclerosing stromal tumors (GIST tumorlets) are common in adults and frequently show c-KIT mutations. Am J Surg Pathol 31:113-120
2. Nilsson B, Bumming P, Meis-Kindblom JM et al (2005) Gastrointestinal stromal tumors: the incidence, prevalence, clinical course, and prognostication in the pre-imatinib mesylate era-a population-based study in western Sweden. Cancer 103:821–829
3. Miettinen M, Lasota J (2006) Gastrointestinal stromal tumors: pathology and prognosis at different sites. Semin Diagn Pathol 23:70–78
4. Gold JS, Gonen M, Gutierrez A et al (2009) Development and validation of a prognostic nomogram for recurrence-free survival after complete surgical resection of localized primary gastrointestinal stromal tumor: a retrospective analysis. Lancet Oncol 10:1045–1052
5. Plaat BE, Hollema H, Molenaar WM et al (2000) Soft tissue leiomyosarcomas and malignant gastrointestinal stromal tumors: differences in clinical outcome and expression of multidrug resistance proteins. J Clin Oncol 18:3211-3220
6. de Pas T, Casali PG, Toma S et al; Italian Sarcoma Group (2003) Gastrointestinal stromal tumors: should they be treated with the same systemic chemotherapy as other soft tissue sarcomas? Oncology 64:186-188
7. Hirota S, Isozaki K, Moriyama Y et al (1998) Gain-of-function mutations of c-kit in human gastrointestinal stromal tumors. Science 279:577–580
8. Heinrich MC, Corless CL, Duensing A et al (2003) PDGFRA activating mutations in gastrointestinal stromal tumors. Science 299:708–710
9. Joensuu H, Roberts PJ, Sarlomo-Rikala M et al (2001) Effect of the tyrosine kinase inhibitor STI571 in a patient with a metastatic gastrointestinal stromal tumor. N Engl J Med 344:1052-1056
10. Verweij J, Casali PG, Zalcberg J et al (2004) Progression-free survival in gastrointestinal stromal tumours with high-dose imatinib: randomised trial. Lancet 364:1127-1134
11. Blanke CD, Rankin C, Demetri GD et al (2008) Phase III randomized, intergroup trial assess-

ing imatinib mesylate at two dose levels in patients with unresectable or metastatic gastrointestinal stromal tumors expressing the kit receptor tyrosine kinase: S0033. J Clin Oncol 26:626–632

12. Heinrich MC, Corless CL, Demetri GD et al (2003) Kinase mutations and imatinib response in patients with metastatic gastrointestinal stromal tumor. J Clin Oncol 21:4342-4349

13. Wang JH, Lasota J, and Miettinen M (2011) Succinate Dehydrogenase subunit B (SDHB) is expressed in neurofibromatosis 1-associated gastrointestinal stromal tumors (GISTs): implications for the SDHB expression based classification of GISTs. J Cancer 2:90-93

14. The NCCN soft tissue sarcoma clinical practice guidelines in oncology (version 1, 2010) (c) 2010 National Comprehensive Cancer Network, Inc. To view the most recent and complete version of the guideline, go online to www.nccn.org 2010. http://www.nccn.org

15. Casali PG, Blay JY; ESMO/CONTICANET/EUROBONET Consensus Panel of Experts (2010) Gastrointestinal stromal tumours: ESMO clinical practice Guidelines for diagnosis, treatment and follow-up. Ann Oncol 21 Suppl 5:v98-102

16. Hohenberger P, Ronellenfitsch U, Oladeji O et al (2010) Pattern of recurrence in patients with ruptured primary gastrointestinal stromal tumour. Br J Surg 97:1854–1859

17. Fiore M, Palassini E, Fumagalli E et al (2009) Preoperative imatinib mesylate for unresectable or locally advanced primary gastrointestinal stromal tumors (GIST). Eur J Surg Oncol 35:739-745

18. Raut CP, Posner M, Desai J et al (2006) Surgical management of advanced gastrointestinal stromal tumors after treatment with targeted systemic therapy using kinase inhibitors. J Clin Oncol 24:2325-2331

19. DeMatteo RP, Maki RG, Singer S et al (2007) Results of tyrosine kinase inhibitor therapy followed by surgical resection for metastatic gastrointestinal stromal tumor. Ann Surg 245:347-352

20. Gronchi A, Fiore M, Miselli F et al (2007) Surgery of residual disease following molecular-targeted therapy with imatinib mesylate in advanced/metastatic GIST. Ann Surg 245:341-346

21. Gramza AW, Corless CL, Heinrich MC (2009) Resistance to tyrosine kinase Inhibitors in gastrointestinal stromal tumors. Clin Cancer Res 15:7510-7518

22. Dematteo RP, Ballman KV, Antonescu CR et al (2009) Adjuvant imatinib mesylate after resection of localised, primary gastrointestinal stromal tumour: a randomised, double-blind, placebo-controlled trial. Lancet 373:1097–104

23. Joensuu H, Eriksson M, Hatrmann J et al (2011) Twelve versus 36 months of adjuvant imatinib (IM) as treatment of operable GIST with a high risk of recurrence: final results of a randomized trial (SSGXVIII/AIO). J Clin Oncol 29: (suppl; abstr LBA1) 2011 ASCO Annual Meeting

24. Gastrointestinal Stromal Tumor Meta-Analysis Group (MetaGIST) (2010) Comparison of two doses of imatinib for the treatment of unresectable or metastatic gastrointestinal stromal tumors: a meta-analysis of 1,640 patients. J Clin Oncol 28:1247-1253

25. Zalcberg JR, Verweij J, Casali PG et al, EORTC Soft Tissue and Bone Sarcoma Group, the Italian Sarcoma Group; Australasian Gastrointestinal Trials Group (2005) Outcome of patients with advanced gastro-intestinal stromal tumours crossing over to a daily imatinib dose of 800 mg after progression on 400 mg. Eur J Cancer 41:1751-1757

26. Demetri GD, van Oosterom AT, Garrett CR et al (2006) Efficacy and safety of sunitinib in patients with advanced gastrointestinal stromal tumour after failure of imatinib: a randomised controlled trial. Lancet 368:1329–1338

27. George S, Blay JY, Casali PG et al (2009) Clinical evaluation of continuous daily dosing of sunitinib malate in patients with advanced gastrointestinal stromal tumour after imatinib failure. Eur J Cancer 45:1959–1968

28. Schittenhelm MM, Shiraga S, Schroeder A et al (2006) Dasatinib (BMS- 354825), a dual SRC/ABL kinase inhibitor, inhibits the kinase activity of wild-type, juxta-membrane, and activation loop mutant KIT isoforms associated with human malignancies. Cancer Res 66:473–481

29. Wiebe L, Kasza KE, Maki RG et al (2008) Activity of sorafenib (SOR) in patients (pts) with imatinib (IM) and sunitinib (SU)-resistant (RES) gastrointestinal stromal tumors (GIST): a phase II trial of the University of Chicago Phase II consortium. J Clin Oncol 26:553s

30. Mankoff DA et al (2007) Tumor-specific positron emission tomography imaging in patients: [18F] fluorodeoxyglucose and beyond. Clin Canc Res 13:3460-3469
31. Stroobants S, Goeminne J, Seegers M et al (2003) 18FDG-Positron emission tomography for the early prediction of response in advanced soft tissue sarcoma treated with imatinib mesylate (Glivec). Eur J Cancer 39:2012-2020
32. Shankar S, van Sonnenberg E, Desai J et al (2005) Gastrointestinal stromal tumor: new nodule-within-a-mass pattern of recurrence after partial response to imatinib mesylate. Radiology 235:892–898
33. Choi H, Charnsangavej C, Faria SC et al (2007) Correlation of computed tomography and positron emission tomography in patients with metastatic gastrointestinal stromal tumor treated at a single institution with imatinib mesylate: proposal of new computed tomography response criteria. J Clin Oncol 25:1753-1759
34. Le Cesne A, Van Glabbeke M, Verweij J et al (2009) Absence of progression as assessed by response evaluation criteria in solid tumors predicts survival in advanced GI stromal tumors treated with imatinib mesylate: the intergroup EORTC-ISG-AGITG phase III trial. J Clin Oncol 27:3969-3974
35. Desai J (2011) Response assessment in gastrointestinal stromal tumor. Int J Cancer 128:1251-1258
36. Prior JO, Montemurro M, Orcurto MV et al (2009) Early prediction of response to sunitinib after imatinib failure by 18F-fluorodeoxyglucose positron emission tomography in patients with gastrointestinal stromal tumor. J Clin Oncol 27:439-445
37. Lencioni R, Llovet JM (2010) Modified RECIST (mRECIST) assessment for hepatocellular carcinoma. Semin Liver Dis 30:52-60
38. Hong X, Choi H, Loyer EM et al (2006) Gastrointestinal stromal tumor: role of CT in diagnosis and surveillance after treatment with imatinib. RadioGraphics 26:481–449
39. Therasse P, Arbuck SG, Eisenhauer EA et al (2000) New guidelines to evaluate the response to treatment in solid tumors: European Organization for Research and Treatment of Cancer, National Cancer Istitute of the United States, National Cancer Institute of Canada. J Natl Cancer Inst 92:205-216
40. Phongkitkarun S, Phaisanphrukkun C, Jatchavala J, Sirachainan E (2008) Assessment of gastrointestinal stromal tumors with computed tomography following treatment with imatinib mesylate. World J Gastroenterol 14:892-898
41. Benjamin RS, Choi H, Macapinlac HA et al (2007) We should desist using RECIST, at least in GIST. J Clin Oncol. 25:1760-1764
42. Bensimhon D, Soyer P, Brouland JP et al (2008) Gastrointestinal stromal tumors: role of Computed Tomography before and after treatment. Gastroenterol Clin Biol 32(1 Pt. 1):91-97
43. Desai J (2011) Response assessment in gastrointestinal stromal tumor. Int J Cancer 128:1251-1258
44. Menu Y (2007) Evaluation of tumor response to treatment with targeted therapies: standard or targeted criteria? Bull Cancer 94(7 Suppl):F231-9
45. Bensimhon D, Soyer P, Boudiaf M et al (2009) Imaging of gastrointestinal stromal tumors. J Radiol 90:469-480
46. Dudeck O, Zeile M, Reichardt P, Pink D (2011) Comparison of RECIST and Choi criteria for computed tomographic response evaluation in patients with advanced gastrointestinal stromal tumor treated with sunitinib. Ann Oncol 22:1828-1833
47. Mabillea,M, Vanela,D, Albiterd M et al (2009) Follow-up of hepatic and peritoneal metastases of gastrointestinal tumors (GIST) under Imatinib therapy requires different criteria of radiological evaluation (size is not everything!!!)". European Journal of Radiology 69:204–208
48. Antoch G, Kanja J et al (2004) Comparison of PET, CT and Dual Modality PET/CT imaging for monitoring of imatinib (STI571) therapy in patients with gastrointestinal stromal tumors. J Nucl Med 45:357-365
49. Choi H, Charnsangave C, de Castro Faria S et al (2004) CT evaluation of the response of gastrointestinal stromal tumors after imatinib mesylate treatment: a quantitative analysis correlated with FDG PET findings. AJR Am J Roentgenol 183:1619-1628

50. Gayed I, Vu T, Iyer R et al (2004) The role of 18F-FDG PET in staging and early prediction of response to therapy of recurrent gastrointestinal stromal tumors. J Nucl Med 45:17-21

51. Holdsworth CH, Badawi RD, Manola JB et al (2007) CT and PET: early prognostic indicators of response to imatinib mesylate in patients with gastrointestinal stromal tumor. AJR Am J Roentgenol 189:W324-30

52. Prenen H, Stefan C, Landuyt B et al (2005) Imatinib mesylate inhibits glucose uptake in gastrointestinal stromal tumor cells by downregulation of the glucose transporters recruiment to the plasma membrane. Am J Biochemi Biotechnol 1:95-102

53. Cullinane C, Dorow DS, Kansara M et al (2005) An in vivo tumor model exploiting metabolic response as a biomarker for targeted drug development. Cancer Res 65:9633-9636

54. Stroobants S, Goeminne J, Seegers M et al (2003) 18FDG-Positron emission tomography for the early prediction of response in advanced soft tissue sarcoma treated with imatinib mesylate (Glivec). Eur J Cancer 39:2012-2020

55. Goerres GW, Stupp R, Barghouth G et al (2005) The value of PET, CT and in-line PET/CT in patients with gastrointestinal stromal tumours: long-term outcome of treatment with imatinib mesylate. Eur J Nucl Med Mol Imaging 32:153-162

56. Tang L, Zhang XP, Sun YS et al (2011) Gastrointestinal stromal tumors treated with imatinib mesylate: apparent diffusion coefficent in the evaluation of therapy response in patients. Radiology 258:729-738

57. Stroszczynski C, Jost D, Reichardt P et al (2005) Follow-up of gastro-intestinal stromal tumours (GIST) during treatment with imatinib mesylate by abdominal MRI. Eur Radiol 15:2448-2456

58. Schlemmer M, Sourbrona S, Schinwaldb N et al (2011) Perfusion patterns of metastatic gastrointestinal stromal tumor lesions under specific molecular therapy. Eur J Radiol 77:312–314

59. Apfaltrer P, Meyer M, Meier C et al (2012) Contrast-enhanced dual-energy CT of gastrointestinal stromal tumors is iodine-related attenuation a potential indicator of tumor response? Invest Radiol 47:65–70

Renal Cancer

4

Cinzia Ortega, Camillo Porta, Manuela Racca and Filippo Russo

4.1 Introduction

Renal cell carcinoma (RCC) represents 2–3% of all cancers, with the highest incidence in Western countries and particularly in Europe, where the annual increase in the incidence of this disease is 2% [1, 2]. More than 50% of RCCs are diagnosed incidentally and are asymptomatic. The classic triad of flank pain, gross hematuria, and a palpable abdominal mass is seen in very few patients (6–10%). Paraneoplastic symptoms (e.g., hypertension, weight loss, pyrexia, neuromyopathy, anemia, polycythemia, amyloidosis, elevated erythrocyte sedimentation rate, and abnormal liver function) are found in approximately 20–30% of patients with RCC and about 20–30% of all RCC patients have metastatic disease.

RCC comprises mainly four different subtypes that differ both genetically and histologically: clear-cell RCC (cRCC, 80–90%), papillary RCC (pRCC, 10–15%), chromophobe RCC (chRCC 4–5%), and collecting-duct carcinoma (1%). Generally, the RCC types have different clinical courses and responses to therapy. The standard for curative therapy in localized RCC is nephron-sparing surgery. In patients who are not candidates for this surgery due to locally advanced tumor, radical nephrectomy is recommended. Complete resection of the primary RCC either by an open or a laparoscopic procedure offers a reasonable chance for cure.

From a molecular viewpoint, RCC, and especially cRCC, is often characterized by the loss of the von Hippel-Lindau (VHL) tumor suppressor gene. This results in the accumulation of hypoxia inducible factor (HIF)1-α under conditions of normal oxygen tension, in the increased expression of HIF-reg-

C. Ortega (✉)
Division of Medical Oncology, Institute for Cancer Research and Treatment (IRCC), Candiolo (Turin), Italy; Italian Nephro-Oncology Group (G.I.O.N.)

ulated genes, and, ultimately, in the overproduction of several pro-angiogenesis factors, such as vascular endothelial growth factor (VEGF) and platelet-derived growth factor (PDGF) [3, 4]. Another key pathway in the pathogenesis of RCC is the mammalian target of rapamycin (mTOR) pathway, which besides contributing to the regulation of cellular metabolic homeostasis is tightly linked to angiogenesis [3, 5]. This improved understanding of the molecular pathogenesis of RCC, a relatively rare tumor, has provided the rationale for targeting the VEGF/VEGF receptors (VEGFRs) pathway as well as the mTOR pathway in cRCC.

Since 2005, when the results of the sorafenib TARGET trial were first presented at the annual meeting of the American Society of Clinical Oncology (ASCO), seven molecularly targeted agents have proven their activity against RCC within large, randomized, phase III trials: the four multikinase inhibitors sorafenib, sunitinib, pazopanib and axitinib, the anti-VEGF monoclonal antibody bevacizumab (combined with interferon-α), and the mTOR inhibitors temsirolimus and everolimus [1].

Sunitinib, pazopanib, and axitinib are three small-molecule tyrosine kinase inhibitors that act on the intracellular kinase domain of several receptors responsible for tumor angiogenesis and growth, including VEGFRs and PDGF receptors (PDGFRs). These drugs differ primarily with respect to their spectra of kinase inhibition and their relative affinities for each molecular target. Besides VRGFRs and PDGFRs, sorafenib inhibits also the Raf-1 serine-threonine kinase, which is involved in transducing the proliferative signal along the mitogen-activated protein kinase (MAPK) pathway and likely plays an important role in tumorigenesis, cell growth, and cell survival.

Bevacizumab is a humanized monoclonal antibody that directly inhibits circulating VEGF. Despite proving to be active alone in RCC, it has been developed as part of a combination with interferon (IFN)-α, even though the biological rationale for this combination has yet to be fully established.

Finally, temsirolimus and everolimus are two specific inhibitors of mTOR complex 1 (mTORC1), thus blocking, at least in part, the activity of mTOR.

Sunitinib and the combination of bevacizumab plus IFN-α have been tested in phase III trials against IFN-α in a pure first-line setting, whilst temsirolimus has been compared to IFN-α or a combination of the two drugs as a first-line therapy in those patients with disease prognostic features indicating poor risk.

Sorafenib and pazopanib have been compared to placebo in patients pre-treated with cytokines, and in a study made up of patients who were treatment-naïve and those pre-treated with cytokines, respectively, while axitinib has been recently compared to sorafenib in patients pre-treated with sunitinib, bevacizumab plus IFN-α, temsirolimus, or cytokines. In another study, everolimus was compared to placebo in patients pre-treated with either sunitinib, sorafenib, or both.

The results of the registration trials of all these novel agents are summarized in Table 4.1. Based on those results, a temptative treatment algorithm for advanced RCC patients has been designed and is reported in Table 4.2.

Table 4.1 Results of the registration trials of novel agents (from [1])

	Treatment setting	Prognostic groups (MSKCC)	OS (months)	PFS (months)	ORR (experimental arm)
Sorafenib vs placebo	second-line	good: 52% intermediate: 48%	17.8 vs 15.2	5.5 vs 2.8	CR: <1% PR: 10% SD: 74%
Sunitinib vs IFN	first-line	good: 38% intermediate: 56% poor: 6%	26.4 vs 21.8	11 vs 5.1	CR: 0% PR: 31% SD: 48%
Temsirolimus vs IFN	first-line (poor risk)	intermediate: 31% poor: 69%	10.9 vs 7.3	5.5 vs 3.1	CR: 0% PR: 9% SD: 46%
Bevacizumab + IFN vs IFN	first-line	good: 29% intermediate: 56% poor: 8%	23.3 vs 21.3	10.2 vs 5.4	CR: 1% PR: 30%
Everolimus vs placebo	after TKIs failure	good: 29% intermediate: 56% poor: 15%	14.8 vs 14.4	4.6 vs 1.8	PR: 1% SD: 63%
Pazopanib vs placebo	first- and second-line	good: 39% intermediate: 54% poor: 3%	22.9 vs 20.5	11.1 vs 2.8	ORR: 30%

IFN-α, Interferon-alpha; *NA*, not available; *ORR*, objective response rate; *OS*, overall survival; *PFS*, progression-free survival; *TKI*, tyrosine kinase inhibitor; *CR*, complete responses; *MSKCC*, Memorial Sloan Kettering Cancer Center; *PR*, partial responses; *SD*, stable disease.

Table 4.2 Tentative treatment algorithm for advanced clear-cell RCC

Patients		First choice option(s)	Alternative option(s)
Treatment-naive patients	Good or intermediate risk group	Sunitinib or Bevacizumab + Interferon-α or Pazopanib	High dose i.v. IL-2 or Sorafenib (selected patients) or observation (selected patients)
	Poor risk group	Temsirolimus	Sunitinib or best supportive care
Pre-treated patients	Cytokine-pre-treated	Sorafenib or Pazopanib	Sunitinib
	Multikinase inhibitors -pre-treated patients	Everolimus or Axitinib[a]	Another TKI

[a]Not yet registered.

4.2 The Issue of Treatment Outcome Evaluation in RCC

Molecularly targeted agents often cause disease stabilization rather than clear-cut tumor regression; indeed, the response rates observed with the majority of these agents are quite low and cases of CR are exceptional (Table 4.1). Another issue is the frequent induction of intralesional necrosis, an event that not only fails to correlate with a substantial decrease in tumor size, but sometimes even simulates disease progression. This situation was first recognized by oncologists in gastrointestinal stromal tumors (GISTs) treated with imatinib [6]. Finally, ^{18}F-FDG PET, confirmed to be extremely accurate in evaluations of the response to molecularly targeted agents in GISTs (and other solid tumors), has great limitations in RCC.

As a whole, these peculiarities make response evaluation with RECIST extremely tricky [7]. Thus, for all these reasons, response evaluation to molecularly targeted agents in RCC is a rapidly evolving field, and both several alternatives to RECIST and techniques other than CT have been proposed.

4.3   The Choi Criteria and the Modified Choi Criteria

Using contrast-enhanced CT scans, Choi et al. [8] developed novel evaluation criteria to assess the efficacy of imatinib in patients with GISTs. The efficacy of the drug is usually coupled with extensive tumor necrosis, often leading to a paradoxical increase in tumor size and thus to difficulties in response evaluation by established criteria. The Choi criteria include changes in tumor attenuation, expressed in Hounsfield units (HU). According to the authors, a partial response (PR) is defined as a $\geq 10\%$ decrease in 1D tumor size or a $\geq 15\%$ decrease in tumor attenuation on contrast-enhance CT scan, while progressive disease (PD) is defined as a $\geq 10\%$ increase in size without meeting PR criteria by a change in attenuation.

Compared to RECIST, the Choi criteria, which are valid for lesions with a longest diameter ≥ 15 mm, significantly better correlate with the disease-specific survival of patients with GISTs. Accordingly, they have replaced RECIST, at least in the evaluation of these tumors [9]. In addition, the Choi criteria have been tentatively applied also to RCC patients treated with molecularly targeted agents.

In a Dutch study of 55 RCC patients treated with sunitinib [10], the predictive role of the Choi criteria was similar to that of RECIST in the mid- and long-term, whilst they proved to be better at first disease evaluation. Overall, however, the Choi criteria were unable to predict early on which patients would develop disease progression, leading the authors to conclude that these criteria are not likely to change the clinical management of patients treated with sunitinib [10]. Nonetheless, since sorafenib is associated with less tumor shrinkage and greater tumor necrosis (than achieved with sunitinib), other authors [11] wondered whether the Choi criteria could be of greater help in evaluating RCC patients treated with this drug.

Less favorable results were obtained in two other studies, performed in RCC patients treated with a variety of anti-angiogenic agents (including sorafenib), in which the superiority of the Choi (and SACT, see below) criteria over RECIST in RCC were not supported [12, 13].

In the subsequently modified Choi criteria, both the size and the attenuation of target lesions are taken into account in response evaluation. As shown in a study on a small number of RCC patients, the modified Choi criteria are better than either RECIST or the original Choi criteria in predicting time to treatment progression (TTP) [13]. However, these results are preliminary and should be prospectively validated in larger series.

4.4 Optimizing the Threshold of Tumor Reduction: The Thiam Criteria

Starting from the above consideration, that molecularly targeted agents act mainly as cytostatic drugs, Thiam et al. [14] attempted to find a threshold for CT evaluation that better reflects the gain in terms of PFS. Thus, with PFS as the primary outcome, thresholds from −45% to +10% were tested in more than 300 RCC patients treated with sunitinib. A decrease of at least 10% in the sum of the longest diameters was identified as the most accurate threshold to distinguish responders from non-responders. Notably, this study also demonstrated that responders can be identified early on (within the first two treatment cycles) if the novel −10% threshold, instead of the conventional −30% threshold required by RECIST, is applied [14]. Again, however, the results must be confirmed and validated before these criteria can be accepted as a substitute for RECIST.

4.5 Size and Attenuation CT (SACT) Criteria

According to these criteria [12], a favorable response is defined either as a decrease in tumor size of ≥ 20% or a decrease in mean attenuation of ≥ 40 HU at least in one non-lung target lesion, or as a decrease in tumor size of ≥ 10%, and a decrease in mean attenuation of ≥ 20 HU in half of the non-lung target lesions. An unfavorable response is an increase in tumor size of ≥ 20%, or the appearance of new lesions, or a new enhancement in a homogeneously hypo-attenuating non-enhancing lesion, or a change from central necrosis to near complete enhancement of solid portions in the central area of the tumor.

Once again, it is clear that the SACT criteria are not ideal in RCC, since lung metastases, the commonest metastatic lesions in RCC, are not evaluable due to the inconsistent mean attenuation results obtained from averaging between soft tissues and air.

4.6   The Mass, Attenuation, Size and Structure (MASS) Criteria

More recently, the Cleveland Clinic group elaborated a new set of criteria for the evaluation of response to molecularly targeted agents in RCC. The following parameters were considered: mass, attenuation, size and structure (MASS) [15].

Using standard contrast-enhanced CT scans, the authors retrospectively evaluated the response achieved in 84 patients with metastatic cRCC who were on first-line sunitinib or sorafenib therapy. The MASS criteria were thus compared to RECIST, the SACT criteria, and the modified Choi criteria. The objective response to therapy was compared with clinical outcomes including TTP and disease-specific survival.

A favorable response determined according to the MASS criteria had a sensitivity of 86% and a specificity of 100% in identifying patients with a good clinical outcome (i.e., PFS > 250 days) and performed better than either RECIST or the modified Choi criteria. The objective categories of response used by the MASS criteria (i.e., favorable response, indeterminate response, and unfavorable response) differed significantly from one another with respect to TTP ($p < 0.0001$, log-rank test) and disease-specific survival ($p < 0.0001$, log-rank test) [15]. Although clearly promising, the MASS criteria still need to be prospectively validated in larger patient populations [16].

4.7   Going Beyond CT

All the above criteria have been developed using contrast-enhanced CT scans as the standard acquisition technique. Yet, especially in recent years, alternative diagnostic techniques have been developed, including ultrasound, MRI, and PET. New functional imaging technologies allow investigations of changes in tumor neo-angiogenesis during therapy as well as functional rather than strictly morphological evaluation of tumor tissue. The feasibility, accuracy, and reproducibility of these new functional imaging techniques must still be determined. In addition, imaging protocols should be standardized, with respect to the timing of response evaluation, data analysis, and defining the values of the functional parameters used to assess positive and negative responses to therapy. Consequently, functional imaging is still under investigation for response evaluation in metastatic RCC. The reports thus far have been promising but the usefulness of functional imaging modalities in RCC patients awaits both confirmation in a larger patient population and the development of new response evaluation criteria.

4.7.1   Dynamic Contrast-Enhanced Ultrasonography (DCE-US)

DCE-US is able to visualize tumor vascularization and to quantitatively assess the perfusion of a given neoplastic lesion by measuring time to peak intensity and area under the curve (AUC) which correlate with blood flow and blood volume, respectively [17, 18]. The technique requires a phospholipid-based microbubble contrast agent which, remaining confined within the intravascular compartment, enhances the vessel signal and allows detection of blood vessels as small as 40 μm [19].

The Gustave Roussy group first reported the possibility of using this technique to identify patients with RCC who will respond to treatment with sorafenib [4]. Indeed, good responders could be discriminated from non-responders as early as after 3 weeks of therapy, based on the combination of a decrease in contrast uptake > 10% and a stability or decrease in tumor volume [20].

Similarly, among patients treated with sunitinib, in partial responders, defined according to RECIST criteria, the ratio between DCE-US parameters at baseline and on day 15 was significantly different from that of non-responders; furthermore, the peak intensity and the slope of the wash-in significantly correlated with PFS [21].

Presently, a nationwide DCE-US study is being carried out in France with the aim of identifying the best parameters and time points to assess the efficacy of anti-angiogenic therapies in several different solid tumors. The advantages of DCE-US are quite evident: the technique is highly accessible and easy to use, is relatively inexpensive (especially when compared with other imaging techniques), has low inter-operator variability, and can be used whenever necessary without exposing patients to ionizing radiation; in addition, procedure-related adverse events have not been reported [22]. However, DCE-US does have one major drawback, particularly relevant in RCC; it is useless in the evaluation of lesions localized to the lung [22], the most common site of metastases in RCC. Thus, its application is limited almost exclusively to tumors with hepatic, pancreatic, and lymph-node metastases.

4.7.2   Dynamic Contrast-Enhanced Magnetic Resonance Imaging (DCE-MRI)

DCE-MRI is a non invasive method for the diagnosis and staging of cancer. It provides high temporal resolution images on how gadolinium based contrast agents are delivered to the intravascular and extracellular extravascular space (for further details refer to chapter 2). Changes in DCE-MRI parameters, such as K^{trans}, K_{ep} and V_e, may be able to measure tumor response to treatment, and could be particularly sensitive when assessing the new targeted therapies.

Variations in K^{trans}, considered the main imaging biomarker, reflect changes in blood flow, blood volume, endothelial permeability, and endothelial surface area, i.e., the parameters involved in the biological response of the tumor to anti-angiogenic and vascular targeting agents. Most studies accept a change in K^{trans} of > 40% as likely representing a true difference due to a drug effect [23]. In a phase II trial of 17 mRCC patients, sorafenib therapy induced a decrease in K^{trans} of 60.3% [24]. Two different studies showed an association between high tumor K^{trans} before therapy and a prolonged PFS [24, 25].

Another option is to evaluate DCE-MRI data using a semi-quantitative analysis, in particular heuristic parameters, which can be better understood as time/intensity curves. The curve of the change in signal intensity indicates the rate of contrast-agent uptake into tumor tissue and its subsequent washout. The main parameters utilized are the slope of the first pass, the peak of the first-pass curve, and the time to peak. A semi-quantitative approach has been used for tumors of the prostate and breast but must be tested for RCC. However, heuristic parameters are dependent on a wide range of scanning parameters and the reported values are not necessarily comparable among the different anatomic sites.

4.7.3 Diffusion-Weighted Magnetic Resonance Imaging (DW-MRI)

Malignant tissue has a higher cellular density than healthy tissues, resulting in a decreased extracellular space and in lower apparent diffusion coefficient (ADC) values. In tumors, DW-MRI can be used to monitor changes in cellularity over time, and thus tumor response to therapy: an initial decrease in tumor cellularity due to cell death and a subsequent increase in the extracellular space both explain an increase in the ADC. DW-MRI does not require contrast agent administration, is relatively simple to interpret and can be performed rapidly. In addition ADC is a reproducible physical constant that is independent of scanner and operator.

In RCC, the main application of DW-MRI has mainly been in the characterization of primary tumors [26-30]. Recently Desar et al. [31] reported on a preliminary assessment (10 patients) of DW-MRI to evaluate the early vascular effects of sunitinib in patients with RCC. They found a significant increase in the ADC values from baseline after 3 day followed by a decrease to baseline levels at day 10 while no changes were observed in the DCE parameters. Therefore ADC values seem very sensitive to sunitinib induced antiangiogenic effects. Further studies will be necessary to understand if the observed DW-MRI changes may be useful to assess response to target therapy. Thus, as often repeated in this chapter, further evaluations of large series are needed to confirm the utility of the technique, in this case as a reliable examination to identify early responders to targeted therapy.

4.8   Positron Emission Tomography

In RCC, the excretion of ^{18}F-FDG via the urinary tract and the variable potential of kidney cancer (especially cRCC) for metabolizing glucose essentially rule out the use of ^{18}F-FDG PET. Indeed, FDG uptake can range from as low as the background activity to intensely FDG-avid lesions. Consequently, a negative ^{18}F-FDG PET does not exclude the presence of RCC but, on the other hand, a positive scan is fairly conclusive. Thus, in RCC, essentially the only application of ^{18}F-FDG PET has been as a "problem-solving tool" when conventional imaging is equivocal.

When RCC is established to be FDG-avid, PET can be used to evaluate the response to treatment. Kayani et al. [33] investigated the role of ^{18}F-FDG PET as a surrogate marker of response to sunitinib in 44 patients with metastatic RCC. They found that 57% of the patients with cRCC had a metabolic response (> 20% reduction in SUV_{max}) after 4 weeks, but these early changes did not correlate with outcome. Their findings contrast with the initial findings in GISTs, were PFS was longer in patients with a measurable response at ^{18}F-FDG PET [33]. The discrepancy perhaps reflects the inherent biological differences between the two tumor types; 4 weeks may be too early to predict resistance in RCC. In fact, later scans, obtained at 16 weeks, identified a subgroup of patients with increased SUV_{max} and poor prognosis (most of them showing an early metabolic response at the 4-week scan). As commented on by Harrison and George, SUV_{max} represents the tip of an iceberg: when it disappears below the surface of the water, it does not provide any information about the events taking place beneath the surface, but when it rises high above the water's surface it may be more representative of changes going on below [34].

As noted above, when metastatic RCC is not FDG-avid, then there is no role for ^{18}F-FDG PET. Attempts to overcome this problem currently consist of the development of new tracers, for example, ^{11}C-acetate, a tracer of lipid metabolism in the cell membrane that is not excreted via the urinary tract. High acetate uptake in RCC was first reported by Shreve et al. [35] but the efficacy of this tracer in RCC is as yet undetermined, since one study was unable to recommend it for the characterization of renal masses [36] whereas another one did [37]. A recently published case report described an early complete metabolic response to sunitinib in one patient with metastatic RCC, as confirmed by ^{11}C-acetate PET before treatment and 2 weeks after [38]. Nonetheless, a drawback of this tracer is that, owing to its short half-life (about 20 min), its production requires the presence of a nearby cyclotron.

Other tracers can be used to explore different aspects of RCC, such as hypoxic status. Tumor hypoxia, a known factor in poor prognosis and radioresistance, can be noninvasively assessed by ^{18}F-fluoromisonidazole (^{18}F-FMISO)-PET. This tracer diffuses through cell membranes and is reduced when the O_2 partial pressure is < 10 mmHg, such that it accumulates intracellularly; the retention observed after injection reflects cellular hypoxia [39]. Hugonnet et al. [40] used this tracer to evaluate initial tumor hypoxia in 33 patients with metastatic RCC, the related changes after sunitinib, and the possible prognostic value. Up to ten targets were defined by CT before the initiation of therapy, subsequently assessed at 1 and 6 months according to the RECIST criteria. Hypoxia was defined as an SUV_{max} above the mean blood value + 2 SDs and the pretreatment uptake of ^{18}F-FMISO was compared with the uptake at 1 month. The authors found that sunitinib reduced hypoxia in initially hypoxic but not in non-hypoxic lesions. Moreover, patients with initially hypoxic targets had a shorter PFS, although OS was not significantly different.

The newest options lie in directly imaging the molecules involved in the promotion or inhibition of VEGF signaling. Inhibitors of the VEGF pathway, such as the monoclonal antibody bevacizumab, can be simply radiolabeled with positron-emitting radionuclides. The idea of assessing and quantifying the uptake of these tracers by the different tumor types (also through dynamic PET studies) is a very enticing one [22].

A recent study examined the feasibility of using [89]Zr-bevacizumab, measured by PET imaging, as a biomarker before and during sunitinib or bevacizumab plus IFN treatment in patients with RCC. [89]Zr-bevacizumab PET imaging is likely to be a promising biomarker if the treatment target (VEGF) can be visualized and if uptake changes after treatment institution [41] can be visualized. The results of such studies are eagerly awaited.

This targeted approach may improve patient selection and therapeutic management, perhaps even allowing the prediction of tumor response before the initiation of therapy. Radiolabeled targeted agents could prevent unnecessary morbidity and lead to substantial cost savings and, most importantly, better patient outcome. Moreover, they could help to reveal different resistance pathways and, finally, to allow the development of combined treatment schedules [42]. In summary, specific PET tracers could provide a unique means for accurate and personalized treatment planning.

4.9   Conclusions

Among all the challenges posed by molecularly targeted agents with respect to RCC, response evaluation is one of the most important. In fact, to truly exploit the potentials of all these drugs, reproducible and accurate criteria are needed that will allow clinicians to identify patients who will benefit from a particular treatment (and those who will not).

Stopping treatment due to what in reality is an inaccurate evaluation of its effect is clinically irresponsible and dangerous for patients, as is, conversely, the continuation of treatment beyond clinical benefit, especially with all the alternative treatment options that are presently available. Furthermore, the economic burden associated with the inappropriate use of these highly costly drugs must also be considered, especially given the current global shortage of resources. Despite the plethora of novel imaging techniques and response evaluation criteria proposed during the past few years, a consensus on the best one is still a long ways away, underlining the need for urgent prospective studies in this field.

Clinical Case

Case History

A 71-year-old woman with hypertension and pre-existing renal colic underwent left radical nephrectomy for cRCC (Fuhrman type I/IV, pT3a with lung and pancreatic metastases) on May 26, 2007. The patient refused upfront treatment aimed at ameliorating her performance status before medical treatment was started. Her characteristics are reported in Table 4.3. At the start of medical treatment, on August 13, 2007, she underwent a CT scan that showed metastases in the following regions: pulmonary, 6 mm nodule; body and tail of the pancreas, two large hyperdense masses (Fig. 4.1); right adrenal gland; right gluteus, hyperdense nodule infiltrating the muscle and the surrounding fatty tissue.

The patient underwent three-cycles of sunitinib with the standard schedule: 50 mg/day for 4 weeks on/2 weeks off. The treatment was well tolerated as only minor side effects were reported (oral mucositis G1 and rash on the chin and forehead G2 according to CTCAE 4). In January 2008, the patient underwent a follow-up CT scan (Fig. 4.2) and was classified as having stable disease according to the RECIST criteria (sum of the longest 1D diameters from 110 mm to 93 mm; size reduction $\cong$ 15%). In March 2008, the patient stopped sunitinib treatment due to renal failure and underwent dialysis.

Table 4.3 Patient's clinical characteristics

Cardiac evaluation	ECG: sinus rhythm 80/min, normal Blood pressure: 150/90 mmHg Left ventricular ejection fraction on echocardio-Doppler: 60% Initial disturbances of left ventricular relaxation
Symptoms	Epigastric pain with a full stomach and right buttock pain radiating to the lower limb ipsilaterally
Examination	Nothing to report
Blood test abnormalities	Mild anemia: Hgb 10.2 g/dl
Prognostic Motzer score	Intermediate

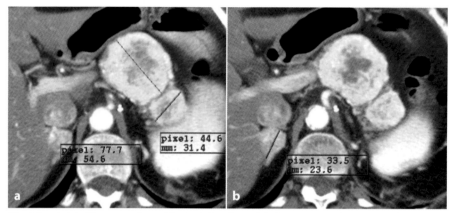

Fig. 4.1 a Axial CT scan performed in the delayed arterial phase shows a large RCC metastasis of the pancreatic body, with the longest diameter measuring 55 mm. A second, 31-mm hypervascular lesion can be appreciated at the level of the pancreas tail. **b** A slightly more caudal scan, passing through the right adrenal gland, shows a third, 24-mm metastasis. The sum of the longest diameters of the three target lesions is 110 mm

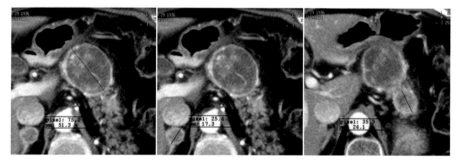

Fig. 4.2 The CT study perfomed after three cycles of sunitinib therapy shows a 15.5% reduction in the sum of the longest diameters of the three target lesions. This case was defined as stable disease according to RECIST, despite the appearance of extensive necrosis within the lesions

Discussion and Conclusion

This case shows the limitations of the RECIST criteria in evaluating response to targeted therapy. Changes in tumor density at CT during anti-tumoral therapy, due to extensive necrosis, is often a remarkable sign of tumoral response; however, it is not recognized by RECIST, in which a partial response is defined as a ≥ 30% decrease in the sum of the longest diameters of the target lesions. Indeed, in the presented case the reduction in diameter compared to baseline was only 15.5% and the patient was classified as having stable disease. However, the association of density and dimensional criteria would have classified this case as a partial response. For example, the MASS evaluation method predicts a favorable response if one of the following findings is

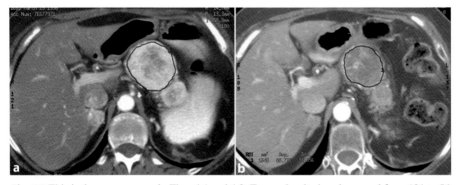

Fig. 4.3 This is the same case as in Figs. 4.1 and 4.2. Tumor density has decreased from 191 to 56 HU between the baseline CT (**a**) and the follow-up (**b**) scan, due to extensive necrosis within the larger lesion. Changes in the density parameters identify this case as a partial response according to the Choi criteria and a favorable response according to the MASS criteria

observed: a decrease in tumor size $\geq$ 20% or one or more predominantly solid enhancing lesions with marked central necrosis yielding a decreased attenuation $\geq$ 40 HU. In our clinical case, the extensive necrosis of the larger lesion compared to baseline (Fig. 4.3) brought about a decrease in density from 191 to 56 HU (69%). Changes in the density parameters identified this individual as a partial responder according to the Choi criteria and with a favorable response according to the MASS criteria.

References

1. Hutson TE (2011) Targeted therapies for the treatment of metastatic renal cell carcinoma: clinical evidence. Oncologist 16 Suppl 2:14-22
2. Ljungberg B, Cowan NC, Hanbury DC et al (2010) EAU guidelines on renal cell carcinoma: the 2010 update. Eur Urol 58:398-406
3. Li L, Kaelin WG Jr (2011) New insights into the biology of renal cell carcinoma. Hematol Oncol Clin North Am 25:667-686
4. Baldewijns MM, van Vlodrop IJ, Vermeulen PB et al (2010) VHL and HIF signalling in renal cell carcinogenesis. J Pathol 221:125-138
5. Wysocki PJ (2009) mTOR in renal cell cancer: modulator of tumor biology and therapeutic target. Expert Rev Mol Diagn 9:231-241
6. Desai J (2011) Response assessment in gastrointestinal stromal tumor. Int J Cancer 128:1251-1258
7. Therasse P, Arbuck SG, Eisenhauer EA et al (2000) New guidelines to evaluate the response to treatment in solid tumors. European Organization for Research and Treatment of Cancer, National Cancer Institute of the United States, National Cancer Institute of Canada. J Natl Cancer Inst 92:205-216
8. Choi H, Charnsangavej C, Faria SC et al (2007) Correlation of computed tomography and positron emission tomography in patients with metastatic gastrointestinal stromal tumor treat-

ed at a single institution with imatinib mesylate: proposal of new computed tomography response criteria. J Clin Oncol 25:1753-1759

9. Benjamin RS, Choi H, Macapinlac HA et al (2007) We should desist using RECIST, at least in GIST. J Clin Oncol 25:1760-1764

10. Van der Veldt AA, Meijerink MR et al (2010) Choi response criteria for early prediction of clinical outcome in patients with metastatic renal cell cancer treated with sunitinib. Br J Cancer 102:803-809

11. Maksimovic O, Schraml C, Hartmann JT et al (2010) Evaluation of response in malignant tumors treated with the multitargeted tyrosine kinase inhibitor sorafenib: a multitechnique imaging assessment. AJR Am J Roentgenol 194:5-14

12. Smith AD, Lieber ML, Shah SN (2010) Assessing tumor response and detecting recurrence in metastatic renal cell carcinoma on targeted therapy: importance of size and attenuation on contrast-enhanced CT. AJR Am J Roentgenol 194:157-165

13. Nathan PD, Vinayan A, Stott D et al (2010) CT response assessment combining reduction in both size and arterial phase density correlates with time to progression in metastatic renal cancer patients treated with targeted therapies. Cancer Biol Ther 9:15-19

14. Thiam R, Fournier LS, Trinquart L et al (2010) Optimizing the size variation threshold for the CT evaluation of response in metastatic renal cell carcinoma treated with sunitinib. Ann Oncol 21:936-941

15. Smith AD, Shah SN, Rini BI et al (2010) Morphology, Attenuation, Size, and Structure (MASS) criteria: assessing response and predicting clinical outcome in metastatic renal cell carcinoma on antiangiogenic targeted therapy. AJR Am J Roentgenol 194:1470-1478

16. Payton S (2010) Kidney cancer: MASS criteria predict good clinical outcome. Nat Rev Urol 7:366

17. Lassau N, Roche A (2007) Imaging and angiogenesis: DCE-US (dynamic contrast enhanced-ultrasonography). Bull Cancer 94:S247-S253

18. Kabakci N, Igci E, Secil M et al (2005) Echo contrast-enhanced power Doppler ultrasonography for assessment of angiogenesis in renal cell carcinoma. J Ultrasound Med 24:747-753

19. Lassau N, Koscielny S, Opolon P et al (2001) Evaluation of contrast-enhanced color Doppler ultrasound for the quantification of angiogenesis in vivo. Invest Radiol 36:50-55

20. Lamuraglia M, Escudier B, Chami L et al (2006) To predict progression-free survival and overall survival in metastatic renal cancer treated with sorafenib: pilot study using dynamic contrast-enhanced Doppler ultrasound. Eur J Cancer 42:2472-2479

21. Lassau N, Koscielny S, Albiges L et al (2010) Metastatic renal cell carcinoma treated with sunitinib: early evaluation of treatment response using dynamic contrast-enhanced ultrasonography. Clin Cancer Res 16:1216-1225

22. Van der Veldt AA, Meijerink MR, van den Eertwegh AJ, Boven E (2010) Targeted therapies in renal cell cancer: recent developments in imaging. Target Oncol 5:95-112

23. Jackson A, O'Connor JP, Parker GJ, Jayson GC (2007) Imaging tumor vascular heterogeneity and angiogenesis using dynamic contrast-enhanced magnetic resonance imaging. Clin Cancer Res 13:3449-3459

24. Flaherty KT, Rosen A, Heitjan F et al (2008) Pilot study of DCE-MRI to predict progression-free survival with sorafenib therapy in renal cell carcinoma. Cancer Biology & Therapy 7:496-501

25. Hahn OM, Yang C, Medved M et al (2008) Dynamic contrast-enhanced magnetic resonance imaging pharmacodynamic biomarker study of sorafenib in metastatic renal carcinoma. J Clin Oncol 26:4572-4578

26. Paudyal B, Paudyal P, Tsushima Y et al (2010) The role of the ADC value in the characterisation of renal carcinoma by diffusion-weighted MRI. Br J Radiol 83:336-343

27. Schoth F, Persigehl T, Palmowski M (2010) Current role and future perspective of MRI for diagnosis and characterization of renal cell carcinoma. Panminerva Med 52:307-318

28. Taouli B, Thakur RK, Mannelli L et al (2009) Renal lesions: characterization with diffusion-weighted imaging versus contrast-enhanced MR imaging. Radiology 251:398-407

29. Pedrosa I, Alsop DC, Rofsky NM (2009) Magnetic resonance imaging as a biomarker in renal cell carcinoma. Cancer 115(10 Suppl):2334-2345
30. Sandrasegaran K, Sundaram CP, Ramaswamy R et al (2010) Usefulness of diffusion-weighted imaging in the evaluation of renal masses. AJR Am J Roentgenol 194:438-445
31. Desar IM, ter Voert EG, Hambrock T et al (2012) Functional MRI techniques demonstrate early vascular changes in renal cell cancer patients treated with sunitinib: a pilot study. Cancer Imaging 11:259-65. PubMed PMID: 22245974
32. Kayani I, Avril N, Bomanji J et al (2011) Sequential FDG-PET/CT as a biomarker of response to Sunitinib in metastatic clear cell renal cancer. Clin Cancer Res 17:6021-6028
33. Prior JO, Montemurro M, Orcurto MV et al (2009) Early prediction of response to sunitinib after imatinib failure by 18F-fluorodeoxyglucose positron emission tomography in patients with gastrointestinal stromal tumor. J Clin Oncol 27:439-445
34. Harrison MR, George DJ (2011). Better late than early: FDG-PET imaging in metastatic renal cell carcinoma. Clin Cancer Res 17:5841-5843
35. Shreve P, Chiao PC, Humes HD et al (1995) Carbon-11-acetate PET imaging in renal disease. J Nucl Med 36:1595-1601
36. Kotzerke J, Linne C, Meinhardt M et al (2007) [1-(11)C]acetate uptake is not increased in renal cell carcinoma. Eur J Nucl Med Mol Imaging 34:884-888
37. Oyama N, Okazawa H, Kusukawa N et al (2009) 11C-Acetate PET imaging for renal cell carcinoma. Eur J Nucl Med Molec Imag 36:422-427
38. Maleddu A, Pantaleo MA, Castellucci P et al (2009) 11C-acetate PET for early prediction of sunitinib response in metastatic renal cell carcinoma. Tumori 95:382-384
39. Lee ST, Scott AM (2007) Hypoxia positron emission tomography imaging with 18F-fluoromisonidazole. Semin Nucl Med 37:451-546
40. Hugonnet F, Fournier L, Medioni J et al (2011) Metastatic renal cell carcinoma: relationship between initial metastasis hypoxia, change after 1 month's sunitinib, and therapeutic response: an 18F-fluoromisonidazole PET/CT study. J Nucl Med 52:1048-1055
41. Clinical Trial Registration Database. Available from: www.clinicaltrials.gov."89Zr- bevacizumab PET Imaging in Patients With Renal Cell Carcinoma Treated With Sunitinib or Bevacizumab Plus Interferon) a Pilot Study". Registration number NCT00831857
42. Van der Veldt AA, Meijerink MR, van den Eertwegh AJ et al (2008) Sunitinib for treatment of advanced renal cell cancer: primary tumor response. Clin Cancer Res 14:2431-2436

Liver Metastases in Colon Cancer

5

Lorenzo Capussotti, Luca Viganò, Francesco Leone
and Delia Campanella

5.1   Standard of Treatment in Metastatic Colorectal Cancer

Liver metastases are found at diagnosis in up to 25% of patients with colorectal cancer (CRC) and they appear during the first 3 years following diagnosis in another 40–50% [1]. Although liver resection is currently the only therapy producing long-term cure, at diagnosis 80% of patients are not considered to be candidates for resection because of the size, location, and extent of their disease. Radiofrequency ablation has been proposed as an alternative to surgery, but at present its effectiveness in terms of local disease control is still inferior to that of liver resection [2]. Transhepatic arterial chemoembolization (TACE) and transarterial 90Y radioembolization (TARE) are more recent techniques that have been evaluated in patients with locally advanced disease; however only preliminary data are available [3,4] and larger studies are needed to better evaluate these treatments.

In patients with unresectable disease, chemotherapy was long considered to be the sole therapeutic option, but its use was only "palliative" and confined to prolonging survival, albeit for a few months at the most. Fortunately, in the past 20 years, the treatment of metastatic CRC (mCRC) has significantly evolved. Until the mid-1990s 5-fluorouracil (FU) was the only available chemotherapeutic agent with demonstrated efficacy, particularly when modulated by the addition of leucovorin (LV) or folinic acid (FA). However, the low response rate (10–15%) and median survival (10 months) afforded minimal improvement over supportive care. With the introduction of the new cyotoxic agents (irinotecan and oxaliplatin), their combination with FU/FA in FOLFIRI and FOLFOX regimens respectively, and the availability of monoclonal anti-

L. Capussotti (✉)
Surgical Department, Division of Hepato-Bilio-Pancreatic and Digestive Surgery, Mauriziano "Umberto I" Hospital, Turin, Italy

bodies against vascular endothelial growth factor (VEGF) or epidermal growth factor receptor (EGFR), significant improvements in both the response rate and the survival of patients with liver metastases were obtained. These improvements gave rise to a new treatment strategy, in which patients received combined medical therapy and surgery, with subsequent increases in the cure rate.

One of the most relevant of the recent advances in mCRC management, in fact, is the use of chemotherapy to downstage initially unresectable disease, so that a number of patients deemed to have unresectable disease become eligible for potentially curative surgery. Current treatment practice for patients with initially unresectable metastatic disease is to treat with the most effective chemotherapeutic regimen that the patient can tolerate, coupled with surgery that should be performed as early as possible to minimize the side effects of chemotherapy. Liver resection with curative intent can be considered in cases of major response and tumor shrinkage.

Optimization of the preoperative chemotherapy regimen is critical to the success of the curative strategy. In fact, a strong relationship between tumor response rate and resection rates seems evident in mCRC [5]. Currently available strategies aimed at increasing the response rates include the association of the new targeted agents, namely, cetuximab and bevacizumab, and the triple-drug association 5-FU/FA/irinotecan/oxaliplatin (FOLFOXIRI). The latter combination was shown to significantly improve response rate, progression-free survival, and radical surgical resection of liver metastases when compared to the FOLFIRI regimen [6] (Table 5.1).

Two randomized studies demonstrated that cetuximab, a chimeric mono-clonal antibody against the extracellular domain of EGFR, in combination with chemotherapy increases response rates and overall resection rates compared with chemotherapy alone [7, 8]. However, recent insights into EGFR

Table 5.1 Results of first-line treatment studies for metastatic cancer colorectal cancer

Population	Patients (n)	Treatment arms	ORR (%)	R0 (%)	PFS (months)	OS (months)
Unselected	122	FOLFIRI [6]	41.0	6.0	6.9	16.7
Unselected	122	FOLFOXIRI	66.0	15.0	9.8	22.6
KRAS WT	316	FOLFIRI [7]	39.7	2.0	8.4	20.0
KRAS WT	350	FOLFIRI + Cetuximab	57.3	5.1	9.9	23.5
KRAS WT	97	FOLFOX [8]	34.0	4.1	7.2	18.5
KRAS WT	82	FOLFOX + Cetuximab	57.3	9.8	8.3	22.8
Unselected	701	FOLFOX/XELOX [13]	47.0	4.9	8.0	19.9
Unselected	699	FOLFOX/XELOX + Bevacizumab	49.0	6.3	9.4	21.3

WT, wild type; *ORR*, overall response rates; *PFS*, progression-free survival; *R0*, surgery with no residual tumor after resection; *OS*, overall survival.

biology have demonstrated that the benefit of anti-EGFR is restricted to a subgroup of patients [9]. The most relevant finding has been the identification of the mutational status of the *KRAS* gene, which encodes a G-protein involved in the downstream signaling of EGFR, as a predictor of resistance to anti-EGFR antibodies.

In a recent phase II randomized trial (the CELIM trial) [10], patients with non-resectable liver metastases were assigned to receive cetuximab with either FOLFOX or FOLFIRI. The tumor response rate was not statistically different in the two arms (68% with FOLFOX+ cetuximab and 57% with FOLFIRI + cetuximab) and the R0 resection rates were 38% and 30%, respectively. Although these results can be considered as promising, data on resectability are not easily comparable to those of other series adopting different criteria in the selection of patients for surgery.

Bevacizumab, a humanized antibody targeting VEGF, is an angiogenesis inhibitor that can improve overall survival when combined with chemotherapy as a first- or second-line treatment of patients with mCRC. Clinical trials have shown an established, well-tolerated, and consistent safety profile for bevacizumab in combination with standard chemotherapy. Data from phase II and III trials demonstrated that the addition of bevacizumab to chemotherapy increases the response rates by approximately 10% compared with chemotherapy alone, either with FU/FA or with irinotecan-based and oxaliplatin-based doublets. Bevacizumab is the only biological agent proven to confer an overall survival advantage to first-line chemotherapy with FU/LV and irinotecan in unselected patients with mCRC [11,12]. The international randomized phase III study NO16966 concluded that the addition of bevacizumab to first-line capecitabine and oxaliplatin (XELOX) or FOLFOX significantly prolongs progression-free survival and increases the rates of surgery with curative intent [13].

No direct comparison of cetuximab and bevacizumab has been published so far. Many clinicians prefer using cetuximab in patients with "potentially resectable" tumors expressing wild-type *KRAS* on the basis of a supposed higher response rate with cetuximab-based than with bevacizumab-based regimens. However, this choice is supported only by retrospective cross-study comparisons, and the definite benefit of cetuximab over bevacizumab in this group of patients remains to be established. Moreover, the conventional criteria for response evaluation, primarily based on the change in lesion size during therapy, may underestimate the real effect of combinations of chemotherapy and biological agents, particularly angiogenesis inhibitors. The development of criteria that take into account the morphology and metabolic activity of tumor tissue would improve the description of the response pattern and help to define optimal preoperative treatment.

When patients with initially unresectable disease are treated with preoperative chemotherapy, an area of controversy is whether to treat them until the "maximal effect" is reached or to discontinue chemotherapy once the disease has been reduced to the point at which hepatic resection is feasible. As a general rule, preoperative chemotherapy should be stopped as soon as the disease becomes resectable. In fact, the policy of pursuing the maximal shrinkage raises a number of concerns. First of all, the disappearance of some liver metastases on imaging (up to 9% of patients) is probably due to the loss of sensitivity of conventional imaging, particularly PET and CT, after chemotherapy and to modifications involving both the liver parenchyma and hepatic metastases. However, a complete radiological response of mCRC according to RECIST criteria has been shown to be of limited predictive value for complete pathologic response and disease cure. Adam et al. [14] observed a complete pathologic response in 4% of patients undergoing resection following preoperative chemotherapy but none of these patients had a complete radiological response. Further studies reported discordant data, with residual cancer being present in up to 80% of patients [15,16]. Consequently, in patients in whom liver metastases disappeared at imaging, residual disease should always be suspected and resection of the site of metastases is recommended whenever possible. A second issue against prolonged chemotherapy is its detrimental effect on the hepatic parenchyma. Data indicate that the rate of postoperative complications or hepatic failure is strictly dependent on the duration of preoperative treatment, with a significant incidence after six to nine cycles. Accordingly, early assessment of tumor response is of paramount importance in the preoperative evaluation of metastatic disease. In this context, the integration of morphologic and metabolic parameters, together with the dimensional criteria, is thought to play a crucial role in defining the effectiveness of the treatment.

5.2   Standard Criteria for the Evaluation of Tumor Response to Treatment

Response to chemotherapy is one of the most powerful prognostic factors after liver resection for mCRC. Furthemore, in this setting the RECIST criteria are reliable to evaluate the response of hepatic mCRC to standard antineoplastic therapies [17] (Fig. 5.1). The LiverMetSurvey database (www.livermetsurvey.org), an international registry of liver surgery for mCRC, has shown a direct relation between the 5-year survival rate and the response to treatment, as determined using the RECIST criteria. As of June 2011, the LiverMetSurvey included more than 14000 patients who underwent liver resection, including 4851 patients for whom data on response to preoperative chemotherapy are available. In this large sub-group of patients, the 5-year survival rates after liver resection were 64% for individuals with complete response at imaging, 43% for those with a partial response, 41% in patients with stable disease, and only 25% in those with disease progression.

Progression after preoperative chemotherapy has been historically considered as a sign of aggressive tumor biology and of the impossibility to achieve disease control. In 2004, Adam et al. [18] correlated patient survival to treatment response in 131 patients with more than three liver metastases who

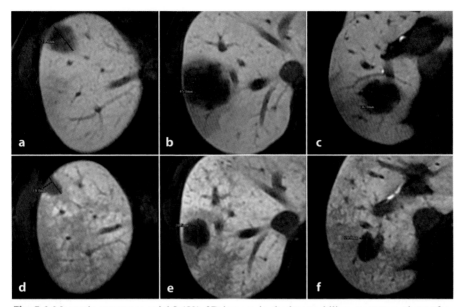

Fig. 5.1 Magnetic resonance axial LAVA 3D images in the hepato-biliary excretory phase after intravenous administration of disodic Gd-EOB-DTPA. Imaging was performed before (**a-c**) and after (**d-f**) chemotherapy. The sum of the largest axial diameters of the target lesions (**a + b + c**) was 110 mm before chemotherapy and 76 mm (**d + e + f**) at the end of the sixth cycle, with a reduction ≥ 30%, thus defined as a partial response according to RECIST criteria

underwent neoadjuvant chemotherapy. Patients with disease progression while on chemotherapy had an extremely poor outcome (8% at 5 years), significantly lower than that of patients without imaging signs of progression. The Memorial Sloan Kettering group reported similar findings in 2007. Dismal survival rates, comparable to those of the untreated patients, led to the decision to consider tumor progression during neoadjuvant chemotherapy a contraindication to liver resection.

Similarly, a pathologic response to chemotherapy was also shown to be associated with prognosis. In 2007, Rubbia-Brandt et al. [19] showed a significant correlation between histologic response, i.e., tumor regression grade, and both overall and disease-free survival in patients undergoing oxaliplatin-based chemotherapy. These data were subsequently confirmed in a series of 305 patients from the MD Anderson Cancer Center who underwent resection and were treated preoperatively with irinotecan- or oxaliplatin-based chemotherapy. In their 2008 study, Adam et al. [14] reported an uncommonly high survival rate of 76% at 5 years in a group of 29 patients with complete pathologic response.

^{18}F-FDG PET was initially introduced in the preoperative staging of CRC to select patients for curative hepatic resection. The use of this imaging modal-

ity resulted in a significant improvement in the survival rates of the surgical patients [20, 21]. Conversely, the role of ^{18}F-FDG PET in the evaluation of response to treatment in the neoadjuvant chemotherapy setting is not yet established. ^{18}F-FDG PET has been incorporated in the revised tumor response criteria for lymphoma, the PERCIST criteria; however, its use in assessing solid tumors, including hepatic mCRC, is limited by availability and cost, in addition to poor spatial resolution and the inability to obtain a precise anatomical localization of the tumor(s). False-negative (e.g., small lesions, mucinous cancers) and false-positive (e.g., normal structures, inflammatory and infectious pathological findings) findings on PET also limit its overall accuracy [22,23].

Lubezky et al. [23] compared the sensitivity and specificity of CT and ^{18}F-FDG PET, using the histopathological reports as reference standard, in two groups of patients: those in group 1 had a total of 33 hepatic mCRC and underwent immediate liver resection; those in group 2 had a total of 122 lesions and received neoadjuvant chemotherapy before undergoing liver resection. In the study, ^{18}F-FDG PET had a lower sensitivity than achieved with contrast-enhanced CT in detecting colorectal metastases following neoadjuvant treatment (49 vs. 65.3%, respectively; $p < 0.0001$). Furthermore, the sensitivity of ^{18}F-FDG PET following neoadjuvant therapy was significantly lower than that determined in patients who did not receive neoadjuvant treatment (49 vs. 93.3% respectively; $p < 0.0001$). Lesion size was one of the main determinants for the decreased sensitivity of ^{18}F-FDG PET. Lubezky et al. [23] also reported an overall specificity of only 83% for ^{18}F-FDG PET; furthermore, in the group of patients receiving neoadjuvant chemotherapy following liver resection the specificity was even lower (60%). In most cases, the source of false-positive findings at ^{18}F-FDG PET was the presence of granulomatous lesions with a high FDG uptake.

5.3   Experimental Imaging Methods in the Evaluation of Response to Treatment

Recently, evidence has emerged that CT attenuation and lesion morphology, variations of the enhancement patterns following bolus injection of contrast agents, and signal-intensity modifications on different magnetic resonance (MRI) sequences might be better predictors of tumor response to therapy than RECIST [24]. In particular, the new imaging markers could be more effective in evaluating response to targeted agents and to transarterial treatments such as TACE and TARE. With the latter therapies, stable lesion size does not necessarily signify that treatment has failed. Indeed, a reduction of vital tumor tissue could be well evaluated based on changes in tumor morphology and contrast-enhancement patterns.

Chun et al. [25] introduced new morphological criteria to evaluate the response of liver metastases to treatment with targeted agents. According to morphology, each lesion was assigned to one of three groups: group 3 metastases were characterized by heterogeneous attenuation and a thick, poorly defined tumor–liver interface; group 1 metastases were characterized by a homogeneous low-attenuation with a thin, sharply defined tumor–liver interface; group 2 metastases were characterized by a morphology that could not be rated as belonging to group 3 or group 1. Lesions with an enhancing rim were classified in group 3 and resolution of the enhancement led to a group 1 classification. Morphologic response criteria were defined as *optimal* if the lesions switched from group 3 or 2 to group 1, *incomplete* if they switched from group 3 to group 2, and *no response* if the group was unchanged or if it increased. The authors compared both the new morphologic criteria and RECIST with survival in patients who underwent liver resection and in those who did not. Among the 82 patients with stage IV CRC who were treated with a bevacizumab-containing regimen, those with an optimal response by morphologic criteria had significantly better overall survival than those with incomplete or no response ($p = 0.009$); in contrast, response as determined by RECIST was not associated with an improvement in overall survival ($p = 0.45$).

These results suggested that morphologic response is a useful, non-invasive surrogate marker of pathologic response in patients with hepatic mCRC treated with a bevacizumab-containing regimen and that it may provide complementary information to traditional size-based criteria in assessing the CT response to therapy.

A year later, Tochetto et al. [26] compared variations of different CT parameters (maximum cross-sectional diameter, volume, and attenuation) to changes in tumor metabolic activity as measured by ^{18}F-FDG PET in 74 patients with hepatic mCRC treated with 90Y TARE. CT attenuation was the marker that best identified responder and non-responder lesions. Per lesion, the percentage change in the SUV_{max} between the pre and post-treatment evaluation correlated significantly with the percentage change in attenuation at CT ($r = 0.61, P < 0.001$). Based on a >15% decrease in attenuation as cutoff value for response, attenuation was the radiologic criterion that best separated responders from non-responders and was more sensitive and accurate (sensitivity 84.2%, specificity 83.3, PPV 84.2%, NPV 83.3%) than size criteria in helping to predict changes in metabolic activity at ^{18}F-FDG PET following treatment. If this finding is confirmed, CT attenuation changes could eventually be adopted as a surrogate marker for the assessment of response to 90Y TARE of hepatic mCRC.

RECIST has other limitations. As measurable changes in the size of CRC metastases may become apparent only after several months, at the middle or end of a course of treatment, RECIST is probably not adequate either to identify early response or to predict response to treatment in the mCRC model. Early treatment assessment and the prediction of treatment response would allow patient-tailored tumor therapy, thus avoiding ineffective treatments and minimizing unnecessary toxicity and expenses.

MRI may yield potentially useful information in the assessment of early response to treatment. The apparent diffusion coefficient (ADC, also see

Chapter 2) has shown promise in measuring early changes in neoplastic tissue following the initiation of chemotherapy in tumors of different organs. In particular, it is widely known that tumor ADC values increase following successful treatment, reflecting a reduction in cellular density and of barriers to water motion. Increases in ADC values may occur hours to days after the beginning of treatment and prior to changes in tumor size. This suggests that an increase in ADC is associated with treatment-induced tumor regression, such as necrosis [28].

These results were noted also in hepatic metastases as a response to chemotherapy [29-31]. Cui et al. [29] measured the ability of the ADC to predict the response to chemotherapy in patients with liver metastasis from CRC and gastric cancer. After the patients had undergone 42 days of chemotherapy, the authors classified 87 metastases into responding (38) and non-responding (49) according to RECIST. Lesion changes were monitored by means of DW-MRI and largest lesion diameter, both at an early stage (days 3 and 7) and at the end of treatment. While in the early stage the mean maximum diameter was similar to pretreatment size in both groups, the ADC values in the two groups were significantly different ($p = 0.002$); only in the responding group was a robust, early increase in ADC observed. The mean percentage ADC change was significantly different in the two groups ($p < 0.001$) being higher in responding than in non-responding lesions (day 3, 25.4 vs. 7.2%; day 7, 26.2 vs. 9.7%). This study shows that ADC may help to predict the early response to chemotherapy. Similar results have been reported in other studies in which patients with hepatic mCRC underwent less conventional treatments, such as hepatic arterial infusion chemotherapy and selective internal radiotherapy [30-32]. The timing of tumor response evaluation as well as the dependence of measurements on the type of MRI scanner and the type of treatment are key issues that need further assessment before ADC changes can be introduced into clinical practice or clinical trials as a predictor of early response to treatment.

As anticipated, RECIST also underestimates tumor response to the new targeted therapies, i.e., drugs directed at specific targets of the tumor-cell life cycle, such as bevacizumab, as these act primarily by cytostatic rather than by cytotoxic effects and may stabilize or increase tumor size despite an excellent clinical response. The functional alterations induced in mCRC by these therapies (e.g., vasculature normalization, increased necrosis) anticipate the anatomic changes such that conventional imaging biomarkers, which are based on size-related criteria, become suboptimal or non-applicable in the evaluation of treatment response. Perfusion imaging may provide a quantitative and reproducible evaluation of the functional changes occurring inside liver metastases in response to therapy [17].

It is widely known that the efficacy of chemotherapy depends on how well the drugs are delivered to the tumor. Delivery is strictly dependent on the tumor vasculature, the uptake and retention of the drug in tumor cells, the efficiency of metabolic activation of the prodrugs, the intrinsic chemosensitivity of tumor cells, and finally the catabolism and excretion of the drugs. Capillary perfusion and vessel permeability can be measured in vivo by dynamic contrast-enhanced MRI (DCE-MRI) following a bolus injection of a gadolinium-based contrast agent.

Pharmacokinetic analysis of DCE-MRI data yields parameters that describe blood entry and exit from the tissues, such as blood flow, permeability, and the total surface area (K^{trans}, k_{ep} and v_e). Virens et al. [33] did not observe a relation between DCE-MRI parameters, tumor metabolic response on dynamic ^{18}F-FGD PET, and survival in patients receiving cytotoxic treatment. However, in a patient with hepatic mCRC under FOLFOX4 combined with bevacizumab, the same authors [34] were able to show a significant decrease in K^{trans} and k_{ep} that related well with the decreased uptake at ^{18}F-FDG PET but not with RECIST, which showed stable disease.

Recently, Hirashima et al. [35] evaluated the role of pharmacokinetic parameters as surrogate biomarkers of antitumor effects in a phase II trial in which bevacizumab plus FOLFIRI was administered to patients with mCRC. Both quantitative and semi-quantitative parameters (K^{trans}, K_{ep}, AUC_{90} and AUC_{180}) were shown to decrease during treatment and the reduction was proportional to tumor shrinkage (all $p < 0.0001$). Changes in K^{trans} and K_{ep} were detected as early as day 7. Finally, using multivariate analysis, the authors showed a relation between K^{trans} and AUC_{180} and time to progression (K^{trans}: $p = 0.001$; AUC_{180}: $p = 0.024$). They concluded that changes in DCE-MRI parameters are useful pharmacodynamic biomarkers for the evaluation of bevacizumab regimens and that they may predict response and prognosis.

5.4   Conclusions

In the future, criteria for the assessment of tumor response will have to integrate size measurements with the morphologic and functional characteristics of the tumors. The focus should be more on the development of methods to measure tumor response rather than simply on how to measure tumors. This is very apparent in the liver model, particularly after the advent of targeted therapies and of the more advanced transarterial treatments. Functional and molecular imaging has the potential to revolutionize oncological imaging, including monitoring during chemotherapy of hepatic mCRC.

Clinical Case

A 56-year-old woman was admitted to our hospital with severe abdominal pain and vomiting. Ultrasonography revealed multiple liver metastases; a CT scan of the thorax and abdomen showed circumferential thickening of the descending colon (Fig. 5.2a), omental nodes (Fig. 5.2b), and multiple bilateral hepatic lesions (Fig. 5.3a–c). Colonoscopy confirmed a stenosing lesion of the descending colon. At histology, the tumor was classified as a well-differentiated adenocarcinoma of *KRAS* wild-type.

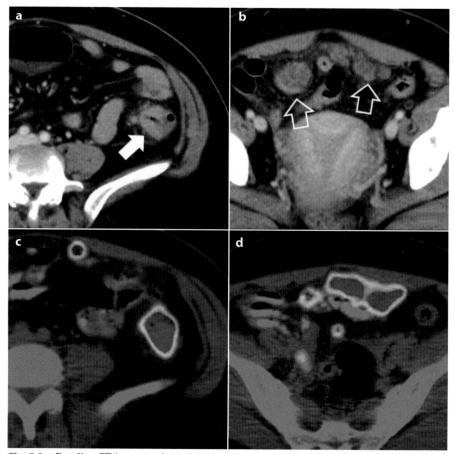

Fig. 5.2 a Baseline CT image performed during the portal phase shows circumferential thickening of the descending colon (*white arrow*), perilesional stranding, and slightly enlarged regional nodes. **b** Multiple omental nodes can be appreciated in a more caudal scan (*open arrows*). **c** Bowel and **d** omental lesions show very high FDG uptake

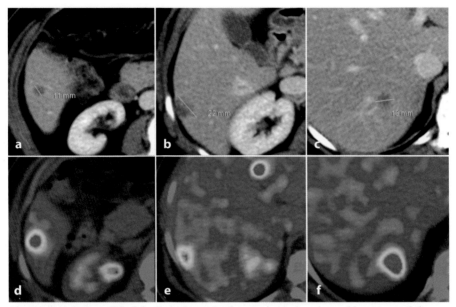

Fig. 5.3 Portal phase CT of the liver shows the three target lesions located in segment 6 (largest axial diameter **a** 11 mm and **b** 22 mm) and segment 7 (**c** largest axial diameter 13 mm). All lesions are slightly hypodense, with ill-defined margins. **d–f** ^{18}F-FDG PET shows abnormal uptake of all target lesions

Laboratory tests revealed normal values of serum bilirubin, transaminase, alkaline phosphatase, and gammaglutamyl-transpeptidase. Total protein levels, prothrombin time, and hemocytometry were also normal. Serological markers were not increased (Ca 19-9: 33 UI/ml and CEA: 2.3 ng/ml).

Total-body ^{18}F-FDG PET showed abnormal uptake in the descending colon, peritoneum (Fig. 5.2c, d) and liver (Fig. 5.3d-f), confirming the diagnosis of metastatic colon cancer.

The patient underwent cecostomy to obviate the bowel obstruction, followed 3 weeks later by systemic therapy with FOLFIRI + bevacizumab. After five cycles, disease restaging with CT showed a significant reduction of the omental findings and a reduction of the bowel-wall thickening (Fig. 5.4a, b) while the hepatic lesions were stable or slightly increased in size (Fig. 5.5a–c). ^{18}F-FDG PET, however, showed a partial metabolic response of all lesions, including the hepatic metastases (Figs. 5.4c-d and 5.5d-f).

A multidisciplinary team consisting of surgeons, medical oncologists, and nuclear medicine and radiology specialists reviewed the patient's medical history and imaging and decided to consider surgical resection pending the results of MRI with liver-specific contrast agent. MRI confirmed all liver metastases previously detected by CT and one additional 6-mm lesion (Fig. 5.6).

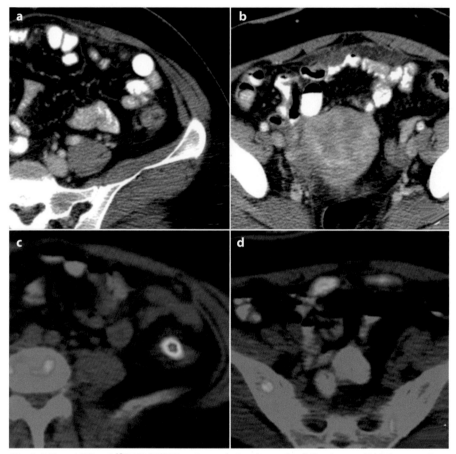

Fig. 5.4 Portal CT and ^{18}F-FDG PET performed after 4 months, following medical therapy, show a significant size reduction of the bowel-wall lesion (**a**) and the omental metastases (**b**). **c, d** The findings are confirmed by a significant reduction in lesion uptake

Following MRI, the patient underwent left hemicolectomy, multiple hepatic atypical resections, partial peritonectomy, and omentectomy. Her postoperative course was uneventful and she was discharged on day 15. Following surgery, she received six cycles of chemotherapy with FOLFIRI regimen and was disease free at follow-up CT performed after 5 months.

This is an example of how the RECIST criteria may be misleading. Measurement of the largest diameter would have classified the liver disease as stable. However, both ^{18}F-FDG PET uptake and lesion enhancement decreased significantly following therapy. In this example, the PERCIST and Choi criteria were more accurate.

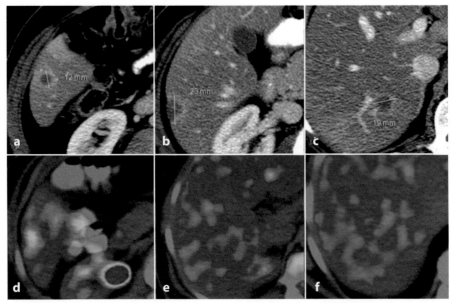

Fig. 5.5 Four months after baseline CT, the three target hepatic lesions are stable (**a, b**) or slightly increased (**c**) in size. They appear markedly hypodense, with a thin peripheral rim of contrast enhancement and sharper margins. While CT showed findings compatible with stable disease according to RECIST, PET/CT demonstrated a complete response in two of the three target lesions (**e, f**)

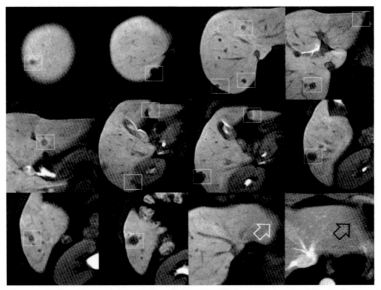

Fig. 5.6 Before liver surgery, MR axial LAVA 3D images acquired in the hepato-biliary excretory phase after the i.v. administration of disodium Gd-EOB-DTPA show all 15 metastases previously detected by CT (*white boxes*) and, in segment 2, an additional lesion of 6 mm (*white open arrow*) not seen at restaging CT (*black open arrow*)

References

1. Jaeck D, Bachellier F, Guiguet M et al (1997) Long term survival following resection of colorectal metastases. Br J Surg 84:977-980
2. Hompes D, Prevoo W, Ruers T (2011) Radiofrequency ablation as a treatment tool for liver metastases of colorectal origin. Cancer Imaging 11:23-30
3. Aliberti C, Fiorentini G, Muzzio PC et al (2011) Trans-arterial chemoembolization of metastatic colorectal carcinoma to the liver adopting DC Bead®, drug-eluting bead loaded with irinotecan: results of a phase II clinical study. Anticancer Res 31:4581-4587
4. Bester L, Meteling B, Pocock N et al (2012) Radioembolization versus standard care of hepatic metastases: comparative retrospective cohort study of survival outcomes and adverse events in salvage patients. J Vasc Interv Radiol 23:96-105
5. Folprecht G, Grothey A, Alberts S et al (2005) Neoadjuvant treatment of unresectable colorectal liver metastases: correlation between tumor response and resection rates. Ann Oncol 16:1311-1319
6. Falcone A, Ricci S, Brunetti I et al (2007) Phase III trial of infusional fluorouracil, leucovorin, oxaliplatin, and irinotecan (FOLFOXIRI) compared with infusional fluorouracil, leucovorin, and irinotecan (FOLFIRI) as first-line treatment for metastatic colorectal cancer: the Gruppo Oncologico Nord Ovest. J Clin Oncol. 25:1670-1676
7. Van Cutsem E, Köhne CH, Hitre E et al (2009) Cetuximab and chemotherapy as initial treatment for metastatic colorectal cancer. N Engl J Med. 360:1408-1417
8. Bokemeyer C, Bondarenko I, Makhson A et al (2009) Fluorouracil, leucovorin, and oxaliplatin with and without cetuximab in the first-line treatment of metastatic colorectal cancer. J Clin Oncol 27:663-667
9. Van Cutsem E, Lang I, D'Haens G et al (2008) KRAS status and efficacy in the CRYSTAL study: 1st-line treatment of patients with metastatic colorectal cancer (mCRC) receiving FOLFIRI with or without cetuximab. Ann Oncol 19(suppl):71O
10. Folprecht G, Gruenberger T, Bechstein WO et al (2010) Tumour response and secondary resectability of colorectal liver metastases following neoadjuvant chemotherapy with cetuximab: the CELIM randomised phase 2 trial. Lancet Oncol 11:38-47
11. Kabbinavar FF, Schulz J, McCleod M et al (2005) Addition of bevacizumab to bolus fluorouracil and leucovorin in first-line metastatic colorectal cancer: results of a randomized phase II trial. J Clin Oncol 23:3697-3705
12. Hurwitz H, Fehrenbacher L, Novotny W et al (2004) Bevacizumab plus irinotecan, fluorouracil, and leucovorin for metastatic colorectal cancer. N Engl J Med 350:2335-2342
13. Saltz LB, Clarke S, Diaz-Rubio E et al (2008) Bevacizumab in combination with oxaliplatin-based chemotherapy as first-line therapy in metastatic colorectal cancer: a randomized phase III study. J Clin Oncol 26:2013-2019
14. Adam R, Wicherts DA, de Haas RJ et al (2008) Complete pathologic response after preoperative chemotherapy for colorectal liver metastases: myth or reality? J Clin Oncol 26:1635-1641
15. Benoist S, Brouquet A, Penna C et al (2006) Complete response of colorectal liver metastases after chemotherapy: does it mean cure? J Clin Oncol 24:3939-3945
16. Ferrero A, Langella S, Russolillo N et al (2012) Intraoperative detection of disappearing colorectal liver metastases as a predictor of residual disease. J Gastrointest Surg [Epub ahead of print]
17. Yaghmai V, Miller FH, Rezai P et al (2011) Response to treatment series: part 2, tumor response assessment - using new and conventional criteria. AJR 197:18-27
18. Adam R, Pascal G, Castaing D et al (2004) Tumor progression while on chemotherapy. A contraindication to liver resection for multiple colorectal metastases? Ann Surg 240:1052-1064
19. Rubbia-Brandt L, Giostra E, Brezault C et al (2007) Importance of histological tumor response assessment in predicting the outcome in patients with colorectal liver metastases treated with neo-adjuvant chemotherapy followed by liver surgery. Ann Oncol 18:299-304

20. Ruers TJM, Langenhoff BS, Neelman N et al (2002) Value of positron emission tomography with [f-18]fluorodeoxyglucose in patients with colorectal liver metastases: a prospective study. J Clin Oncol 20:388–395

21. Fernandez F, Debrin JA, Linehan DC et al (2004) Five year survival after resection of hepatic metastases from colorectal cancer in patients screened by positron emission tomography with 18-fluorodeoxyglucose (FDG-PET). Ann Surg 240:438-450

22. Shanbhogue AK, Karnad AB, Prasad SR (2010) Tumor Response Evaluation in oncology: current update. J Comput Assist Tomogr 34:479-484

23. Lubezky N, Metser U, Geva R et al (2007) The role and limitations of 18-fluoro-2-deoxy-D-glucose positron emission tomography (FDG-PET) scan and computerized tomography (CT) in restaging patients with hepatic colorectal metastases following neoadjuvant chemotherapy: comparison with operative and pathological findings. J Gastrointest Surg 11:472-478

24. Suzuky C, Jacobson H, Hatschek T et al (2008) Radiologic measurements of tumor response to treatment: practical approaches and limitations. Radiographics 28:329-344

25. Chun YS, Vauthey J, Boonsirikamchai P et al (2009) Association of computed tomography morphologic criteria with pathologic response and survival in patients treated with bevacizumab for colorectal liver metastases. JAMA 302:2338-2344

26. Tochetto SM, Rezai P, Rezvani M et al (2010) Does multidetector CT attenuation change in colon cancer liver metastases treated with 90 Y help predict metabolic activity at FDG PET? Radiology 255:164-172

27. Pauls S, Gabelmannb A, Heinzc W et al (2009) Liver perfusion with dynamic multidetector-row computed tomography as an objective method to evaluate the efficacy of chemotherapy in patients with colorectal cancer. Clin Imaging 33:289-294

28. Sun Y, Cui Y, Tang L et al (2011) Early evaluation of cancer response by a new functional biomarker: apparent diffusion coefficient. AJR 197:23–29

29. Cui Y, Zhang XP, Sun YS et al (2008) Apparent diffusion coefficient: potential imaging biomarker for prediction and early detection of response to chemotherapy in hepatic metastases. Radiology 248:894–900

30. Marugami N, Tanaka T, Kitano S et al (2009) Early detection of therapeutic response to hepatic arterial infusion chemotherapy of liver metastases from colorectal cancer using diffusion-weighted MR imaging. Cardiovasc Intervent Radiol 32:638–646

31. Wybranski C, Zeile M, Löwenthal D et al (2011) Value of diffusion weighted MR imaging as an early surrogate parameter for evaluation of tumor response to high-dose-rate brachytherapy of colorectal liver metastases. Radiat Oncol 6:43

32. Dudeck O, Zeile M, Wybranski C et al (2010) Early prediction of anticancer effects with diffusion-weighted MR imaging in patients with colorectal liver metastases following selective internal radiotherapy. Eur Radiol 20:2699-706

33. Vriens D, van Laarhoven HWM, van Asten JJA et al (2009) Chemotherapy response monitoring of colorectal liver metastases by dynamic Gd-DTPA - Enhanced MRI perfusion parameters and 18F-FDG PET metabolic rate. J Nucl Med 50:1777–1784

34. Vriens D, de Geus-Oei LF, Heerschap A et al (2011) Vascular and metabolic response to bevacizumab-containing regimens in two patients with colorectal liver metastases measured by dynamic contrast-enhanced MRI and dynamic 18F-FDG-PET. Clin Colorectal Cancer 10:E1-E5

35. Hirashima Y, Yamada Y, Tadeishi U et al (2011) Pharmacokinetic parameters from 3-Tesla DCE-MRI as surrogate biomarkers of antitumor effects of bevacizumab plus FOLFIRI in colorectal cancer with liver metastasis. Int J Cancer Jul 21, 2011. doi: 10.1002/ijc.26282. [Epub ahead of print]

Part III

RECIST and Beyond: Assessing the Response to Treatment in Locally Advanced Disease

Neoadjuvant Therapy in Breast Cancer

6

Laura Martincich, Ilaria Bertotto and Filippo Montemurro

6.1 Background and Clinical Considerations

Neoadjuvant therapy (NAT), often referred to as primary therapy, is a well-established approach in the treatment of early breast cancer [1, 2]. Historically, NAT was initially used in women with locally advanced breast cancer. In this setting it represented the only chance for a patient with an otherwise inoperable cancer of the breast to obtain a tumor regression that made surgery feasible. These experiences in locally advanced tumors suggested that the primary breast cancers regressed frequently and, sometimes, became clinically undetectable during NAT. From locally advanced tumors, NAT was then studied in women with operable breast cancers, in whom it was speculated that anticancer treatment administered before surgery would offer a number of advantages compared to the traditional approach of surgery followed by adjuvant treatments. For example, in animal models, removal of the primary tumor was shown to have a permissive effect on distant micrometastases [3]; consequently, in the interval after breast surgery, micrometastases could grow to the extent that subsequent adjuvant treatments lost their efficacy. When potent chemotherapy agents such as the anthracyclines and, later, the taxanes became available, the rates of tumor regression observed in breast tumors were so impressive that NAT became synonymous with neoadjuvant chemotherapy (NAC). Furthermore, a rationale was established for challenging the traditional post-surgical adjuvant chemotherapy approach based on NAC, with the aim of improving survival. A large randomized trial conducted by the NSABP (trial B-18), considered a milestone in the field, compared four cycles of AC (doxorubicin 60 mg/m^2 and cyclophosphamide 600 mg/m^2) as neoadjuvant or

L. Martincich (✉)
Radiology Unit, Institute for Cancer Research and Treatment (IRCC),
Candiolo (Turin), Italy

postoperative treatment in 1523 women with operable cancer [4]. This trial failed to show any survival advantage in patients receiving neoadjuvant AC compared to those receiving AC as postoperative treatment, but confirmed that the rate of breast-conserving surgery was higher in women receiving NAC with AC, due to tumor downstaging. The results of several clinical trials are now available and, in general, they challenge several of the original assumptions. This, in turn, has generated controversies about the indications, other than tumor downstaging and more breast-conserving surgery, of this approach. A recent meta-analysis of randomized trials comparing neoadjuvant with adjuvant therapies failed to show a survival advantage for the former modality [5]. One relevant observation from the NSABP-B18 clinical trial, which was consistently reported in other NAC studies, was that a pathological complete response (pCR), defined as the complete disappearance of any evidence of invasive tumor at surgery, was strongly associated with a favorable clinical outcome. This relationship makes NAC, and more generally NAT, an attractive platform to compare treatments and to study mechanisms of resistance to anticancer therapies [6]. In fact, in patients with operable breast cancer, clinical trials evaluating the efficacy of an adjuvant, post-surgical treatment require both large samples of patients and long-term follow-up in order to accumulate an adequate number of disease-related events (locoregional tumor relapses, distant metastases, or death) to allow sound statistical analyses. Conversely, the end-point of pCR is obtained in a relatively short time and is measurable in virtually any treated patient. One of the other potential advantages of NAT is the ability to monitor tumor regression during treatment and to interrupt it in the case of no benefit. This has two implications; the first is the option to spare patients the toxic effects of ineffective treatments; the second is the possibilty to select patients for novel strategies to circumvent treatment resistance. In its modern applications, NAT is no longer synonymous with NAC but includes also endocrine therapy, biologically targeted therapies, and various combinations of medical treatments selected on the basis of the patient's characteristics and the biology of the tumor. Regardless of the goals of NAT–from allowing more conservative surgery to detailed investigations into the molecular mechanisms of tumor resistance to biologically targeted therapies – it remains, as it was at the beginning of its history, the paradigm of a multidisciplinary medical approach. Monitoring tumor regression during treatment is one central aspect of the management of patients undergoing any form of NAT. A primary motivation is that, if a strong indication to NAT is tumor downstaging as a strategy to increase breast-conservation surgery, then tumor dimensions before and after treatment will be critical in the decision as to which type of surgery is applicable. Second, clinical response has been shown to predict the likelihood of a pCR in patients receiving chemotherapy-based strategies. Therefore, close monitoring may provide useful information on the final outcome well before the treatment is completed.

6.2 Monitoring Tumor Response to Treatment

The simplest way to measure tumor response in a patient undergoing NAT is by palpation and by means of calipers [7]. More sophisticated approaches include the different diagnostic imaging modalities, and their potential advantages and limitations have been extensively studied [8-10]. Imaging studies in patients undergoing NAT can provide useful information for the surgeon and the oncologist. With regards to surgery, imaging allows an accurate local staging of disease before treament and, similarly, accurate evaluation of the extent of residual disease at the end of treatment. From the oncological standpoint, imaging should yield information on in-vivo chemosensitivity, also following the initial course of therapy. Mammography (MX), ultrasound (US), and magnetic resonance imaging (MRI) are the radiological modalities applied to the evaluation of tumor response [8-10]. While MX and US provide only morphological criteria, MRI may also contribute to functional features. In the preoperative setting, imaging performed prior to NAT should provide information on lesion size and number and on the possible involvement of the skin and chest wall.

After treatment, the imaging objective is to assess tumor response. The RECIST and WHO criteria are used to evaluate the tumor-volume response to NAT based on comparative changes in the maximal diameter and in the bidimensional diameters of the primary lesion, respectively. In both classifications, a complete response describes the disappearance of all known disease. In addition to radiological features, when evaluating response one must keep in mind other aspects, including tumor biology, drugs effects, and risk factors for local relapse after NAT plus conservative surgery [11].

6.3 Imaging

Although MX represents the most cost-effective modality in screening sporadic breast cancer, it is not the modality of choice in the definition of tumor response at the end of NAT. In fact, in both the evaluation of the extent of residual disease and the identification of pCR, the accuracy of MX is approximately 50% [12,13]. MX provides a qualitative assessment of lesion density and imperfect evaluation of tumor size. In the literature, the correlation between mammographic measurements and those defined by pathology ranges from -0.19 to 0.77, depending on breast density [9]. The superimposition of normal glandular tissue on tumor tissue may lead to an inaccurate evaluation of response. For example, the identification of < 50% of the tumor margins before treatment was shown to be one of the most significant pitfalls in assessing tumor response after NAT [14]. Indeed, visualization of residual vital tumor may be obscured by breast density and by fibrosis secondary to chemotherapy [15] (Fig. 6.1).

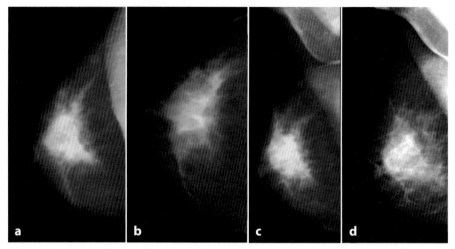

Fig. 6.1 Invasive, lobular, locally advance breast cancer in the right breast, as monitored by mammography. Before treatment, the lesion was visible as an opacity with an irregular shape and irregular margins, as seen on cranio-caudal (**a**) and medio-lateral (**c**) views. The examination performed at the end of treatment (**b** cranio-caudal view; **d** medio-lateral view) showed a reduction in lesion density but due to the superimposition of glandular parenchyma it was not possible to reliably measure the extent of residual disease

Also according to the literature, US is more accurate than MX in the evaluation of breast tumor response to NAT, with values ranging from 43 to 82% [9,16-18]. US is reliable in the measurement of round unifocal lesions undergoing concentric shrinkage. Conversely, it has limitations before treatment, when lesions are characterized by an irregual shape or posterior shadowing, and after NAT, when the lesion fragments and one or more small (< 6 mm) hypoechoic areas with or without shadowing remain [19].

Breast MRI has marked advantages over conventional imaging as it demonstrates both the morphological and the functional features related to tumor neoangiogenesis [10]. MRI provides two types of indicators of response that are relevant to tumor vascularization [9,10]. The first is the morphological variation in tumor size, which, unlike conventional imaging, more correctly analyzes only the vital portion of the tumor based on its vascularity [9,10, 17]. The second is kinetic descriptors of vascular behavior, provided by the signal-intesity/time curves. The absence of enhancement at the site of the previous cancer, a decrease in early contrast uptake, and a flattening of the signal-intesity/time curve are considered indicators of complete response [9,10, 20] (Fig. 6.2). A recent meta-analysis evaluating 25 studies concerning the diagnostic performance of dynamic contrast-enhanced MRI following NAT showed an overall sensitivity for pCR of 63%, which was disappointing [21]. However, the performance was defintely higher than that of either MX or US. In the study of Montemurro et al. [22], a correlation with pathology was much better for MRI than for US with respect to the identification of pCR or small residual

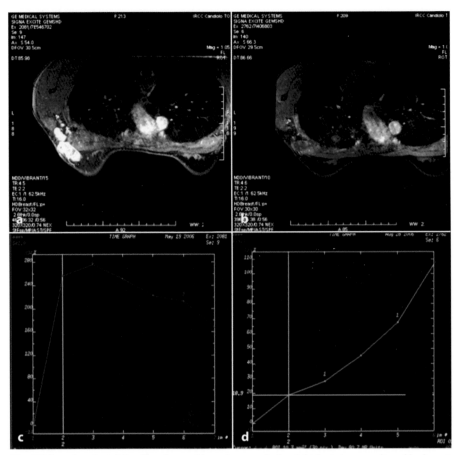

Fig. 6.2 Invasive, ductal, locally advanced breast cancer in the right breast, as monitored by breast MRI. Before treatment, DCE-MRI (**a**) identified an area of mass-like enhancement characterized by an oval shape, irregular margins, and heterogeneous internal pattern in the superior external quadrant. A nodal metastasis was detectable in the ipsilateral axilla. Kinetic analysis of the primary tumor (**c**) showed a strong initial enhancement and a washout signal-intensity/time curve. At the end of treatment, no abnormal enhancement seen either at the site of the primary cancer or in the axillary nodal metastasis (**b**). Kinetic analysis performed at the tumor site (**d**) showed a significant reduction in enhancement and a flattening of the signal-intensity/time curve. The absence of enhancement and the changes in the kinetic features were indicative of a complete response, which was confirmed at pathology

disease (0.731 vs. 0.113, respectively). On the other hand, the specificity of MRI in the identification of pCR was 91% [21].

Several studies have underlined that breast MRI is more accurate than clinical examination, MX, or US in measuring the extent of residual disease at the end of treatment, as it is able to identify changes in the vascular properties of the tumoral bed [9, 10, 21]. The correlation between measurements at pathol-

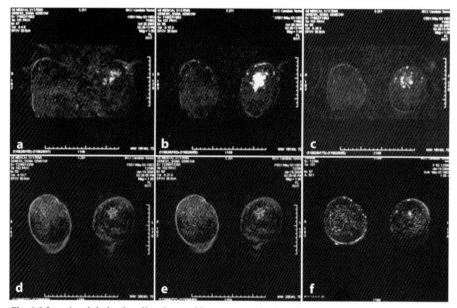

Fig. 6.3 Invasive, lobular, locally advanced breast cancer in the left breast monitored by breast MRI. Before treatment, the lesion was characterized by an irregular shape and heterogeneous enhancement (**a–c**). At the end of treatment, the lesion fragmented and the response was classified as partial (**d–f**). The patient underwent breast-conserving surgery. Pathology showed positive margins because of multiple foci of residual disease < 3 mm in size

ogy and those obtained by MRI ranges from $r = 0.65$ to $r = 0.98$, as reported in the literature [10]. Over- or underestimation of response by MRI occurs in up to 23% of the cases [9, 10, 23, 24]. Underestimation may be due to NAT-induced fibrotic changes since the vascularization of fibrous tissue often resembles that of tumor. While less frequent than in conventional imaging, overestimation may occur in the presence of invasive lobular carcinoma when the lesion has an irregular shape before treatment and when it fragments following NAT (Fig. 6.3).

It was recently shown that MRI visualizes tumor response differently depending on the immunohistochemical subtype of the cancer [25]. Changes at MRI, including DCE-MRI, during NAC correlate well with pathology outcome for triple-negative and HER2-positive tumors, but not for ER-positive/HER2-negative tumors. The reason for this is that triple-negative tumors most often show a unifocal appearance at baseline and undergo concentric shrinkage following treatment. Similarly, HER2-type tumors that present as multifocal masses at baseline may show either concentric shrinkage or no enhancement following treatment. Conversely, no distinctive patterns are appreciated either before or after NAT in ER-positive/HER2- negative tumors.

The technical improvements achieved over the past few years have allowed the application of diffusion-weighted imaging (DWI) to the breast. DWI evaluates the random motion of water molecules in a tissue and provides a functional parameter, the apparent diffusion coefficient (ADC), that is closely related to both tumor cellularity and extracellular water content [26]. DWI does not require contrast agent administration; it has a short acquisition time and allows for rapid post-processing. Furthermore, the ADC is very sensitive to the changes in tumor cellularity and necrosis that occur during anticancer therapy [26]. A recently published study evaluating the role of DWI in assessing tumor response after NAT in 70 patients showed that the overall diagnostic performance of DWI was better than that of dynamic MRI [27]. In the above-reported series, DWI correctly identified eight of nine cases of pCR while dynamic MRI indentified only five of nine. The performance of DWI in assessing non-responder patients was the same as that of dynamic MRI. Even if preliminary, these results suggest that ADC values offer a useful tool in monitoring tumor response to NAT.

Nonetheless, the decision regarding the value of MRI in such cases must be made by the Breast Unit, as thus far there is insufficient evidence from randomized controlled trials that the use of MRI in evaluating the effect of NAT increases the rate of conservative surgery [10]. However, if treatment response is monitored by MRI, then it should at least be performed before the start and at the end of chemotherapy [9,10].

Additionally, MRI studies during NAT may be useful for the early prediction of response. This is a potential field of application of imaging with a more oncological perspective [9,10]. Changes in MRI morphological and functional parameters during NAT were shown to be predictive of response and/or clinical outcome [9, 10], while tumor volume appears to be a reliable early indicator of tumor response. In the series of Partridge and Coll, baseline MRI volume was a strong indicator (more predictive than tumor diameter) of recurrence-free survival, which is related to the achievement of pCR [28]. Tumor volume after two cycles of chemotherapy was associated with a major histopathological response (small cluster of dispersed residual cancer cells or no residual viable cancer cell) at surgery [29]. Changes in uni-dimensional and bi-dimensional criteria during primary chemotherapy were found to be predictive of radiological response at the end of treatment [30]. Changes in the shape of the signal-intensity/time curves were shown to be indicative of pathological response at surgery [31]. More recently, model-based post-processing of MRI data has been applied in the early definition of tumor response. This approach evaluates response to NAT more accurately than non-model-based software kinetics of contrast agents by providing functional parameters (K^{trans}, K_{ep}, and V_p) that better represent the exchange of contrast agent between abnormal tumor vessels and extravascular spaces [32]. In two different studies of Padhani and Coll, changes of K^{trans} during NAT were shown to be a reliable marker in the prediction of response [33, 34].

In this setting, additional MRI techniques (spectroscopy and DWI) are also under investigation. ^{1}H magnetic resonance spectroscopy (^{1}H-MRS) is a non-invasive technique that yields biochemical information in vivo by identifying, in a given volume of tissue, various metabolites, each of which is identified by the position of its chemical shift on a scale of resonance frequencies within a defined spectrum [9,10]. In breast cancer, visualization of the characteristic peak of total choline-containing compounds (t-Cho) at 3.2 ppm is indicative of active tumor [35]. Studies evaluating ^{1}H-MRS (at 1.5T) in the monitoring of patients with locally advanced breast cancer undergoing NAT reported interesting results [36, 37]; however, they also revealed several limitations of the technique that may restrict its widespread use in clinical practice. The main problem was that an absence or reduction of the t-Cho peak during or after treatment may be observed in responders and non-responders. In addition, the long acquisition time (> 10 min) and the need for dedicated post-processing software prohibit the efficient use of ^{1}H-MRS in the clinical setting.

The most encouraging results were reported by Meisamy and Coll [38]. In a preliminary study carried out with a 4T magnet in 16 patients undergoing NAT, they were able to demonstrate significantly different changes in t-ChO between responders and non-responders as early as 24 h after the first dose of chemotherapy. Also, in another study of early response, it was shown that ADC is very sensitive to the changes in tumor cellularity and necrosis that occur during anticancer therapy. Accordingly, DWI was proposed as a promising "biomarker for treatment response in oncology" [39]. High baseline ADC values were predictive of a reduced chemosensitivity in a series of 53 patients [40], while Pickles and Coll found that changes in the ADC values during NAT preceded variations in tumor size [41]. As for ^{1}H-MRS, the evidence from DWI reported in the literature is very preliminary but, as mentioned above, is likely to offer several advantages in future clinical applications.

6.4   Conclusions

In summary, dynamic MRI represents the most accurate modality in the evaluation of tumor response to NAT. The sensitivity of this modality is higher than that of conventional imaging, in both the identification of pCR and the assessment of residual disease extent at the end of treatment. Consequently, it provides more useful information in planning definitive surgical treatment. Hovever, the benefits of monitoring NAT efficacy by DCE-MRI in terms of clinical outcome remain to be assessed. Similarly, the clinical role of emerging techniques, such as DWI and ^{1}H-MRS, has yet to be appropriately evaluated.

Clinical Case

History

A 54-year-old woman presented with a palpable mass in her left breast. She denied a family history of breast cancer. Her health status was good and her past medical history was unremarkable.

On clinical examination, a firm breast nodule was palpable in the upper outer quadrant of the left breast. The main diameter of the lesion, measured by a caliper, was 4 cm and the skin covering the lesion was retracted. At least two enlarged nodes were palpated in the left axilla. Pretreatment imaging of the left breast consisted of mammography and MRI (Figs. 6.4, 6.5).

Apart from the left breast and axilla, her physical examination did not reveal signs of systemic involvement or other remarkable findings. A computed tomography scan of the chest and abdomen did not show lung or liver metastases. A bone scan did not reveal any suspicion areas of uptake. In through-cut biopsies of both the left breast nodule and the axillary enlarged nodes, a G3 infiltrating ductal carcinoma was determined. Immunohistochemistry showed that the tumor was negative for estrogen and progesterone receptor expression. Thr HercepTest score was 1+ (HER2-negative), and the Ki67 score was 70%, indicative of a high proliferative activity.

In summary, this was a cT2, cN2, M0 "triple negative breast cancer." The case was discussed by our multidisciplinary breast team and the decision was made to start the patient on neoadjuvant chemotherapy.

Imaging Before Treatment

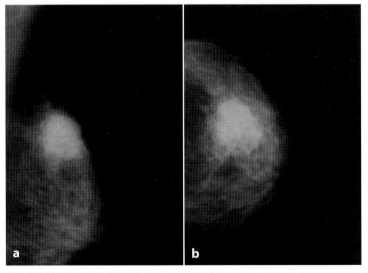

Fig. 6.4 Mediolateral (a) and cranio-caudal (b) views obtained at mammography. A round opacity with irregular margins is visible in the external-superior quadrant of the left breast

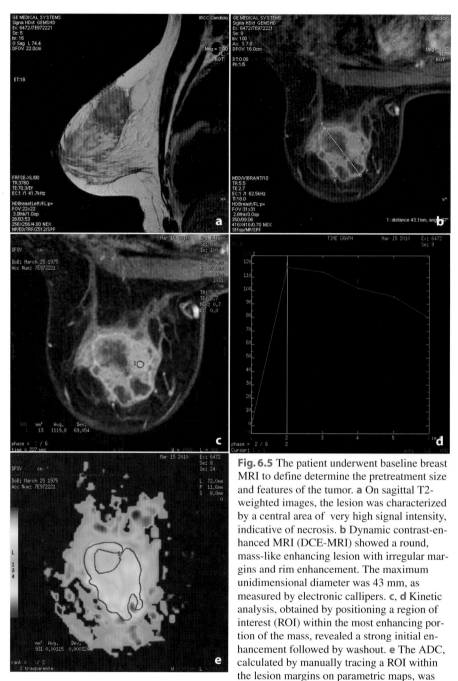

Fig. 6.5 The patient underwent baseline breast MRI to define determine the pretreatment size and features of the tumor. **a** On sagittal T2-weighted images, the lesion was characterized by a central area of very high signal intensity, indicative of necrosis. **b** Dynamic contrast-enhanced MRI (DCE-MRI) showed a round, mass-like enhancing lesion with irregular margins and rim enhancement. The maximum unidimensional diameter was 43 mm, as measured by electronic callipers. **c, d** Kinetic analysis, obtained by positioning a region of interest (ROI) within the most enhancing portion of the mass, revealed a strong initial enhancement followed by washout. **e** The ADC, calculated by manually tracing a ROI within the lesion margins on parametric maps, was 1.15×10^{-3} mm^2/s

Therapy

A 12-lead electrocardiogram and an ultrasonographic evaluation of the left ventricular ejection fraction yielded normal results. Thus, the patient underwent six courses of neoadjuvant chemotherapy consisting of paclitaxel 175 mg/m^2 and epi-doxorubicin 90 mg/m^2, both administered intravenously every 21 days. At each visit, the tumor and axillary nodes were measured with a calipers. During neoadjuvant chemotherapy, both the breast lesion and the enlarged axillary nodes shrank significantly, but a 1-cm, irregularly shaped node was still palpable in the upper outer quadrant of the left breast.

Imaging After Treatment

The breast MRI at the end of the neoadjuvant treatment was indicative of a radiological complete response (Fig. 6.6).

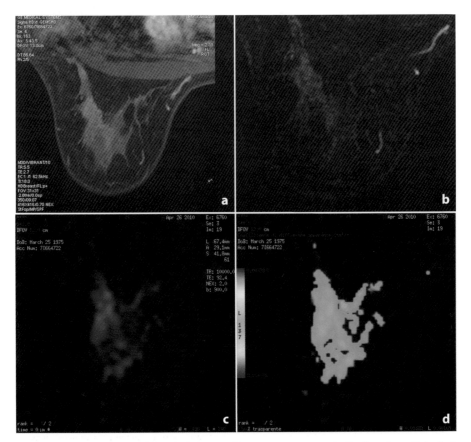

Fig. 6.6 The breast MRI at the end of the neoadjuvant treatment was indicative of a radiological complete response, as no areas of abnormal enhancement or hyperintensity were detectable at the site of the previous cancer. **a** Early post-contrast dynamic acquisition; **b** early subtracted image; **c** diffusion-weighted image acquired with a b-value of 900 mm^2/s; **d** ADC parametric map

Final Considerations

Three weeks after the sixth course of chemotherapy, the patient underwent surgery of the outer quadrant of the left breast and axillary lymph-nodal dissection. The final histopathological report showed the absence of invasive tumor cells both in the breast tissue and in the axillary nodes (pathological complete remission). The patient received adjuvant radiation therapy and underwent regular follow-up controls.

This case shows that MRI can be used to monitor the effect of neoadjuvant chemotherapy, as this imaging modality may outperform clinical examination in predicting a pathological complete remission. By exploiting this ability, physicians will be able to tailor the number of chemotherapy courses according to each patient's MRI response.

References

1. Kaufmann M, von MG, Smith R et al (2003) International expert panel on the use of primary (preoperative) systemic treatment of operable breast cancer: review and recommendations. J Clin Oncol 21:2600-2608
2. Kaufmann M, Hortobagyi GN, Goldhirsch A et al (2006) Recommendations from an international expert panel on the use of neoadjuvant (primary) systemic treatment of operable breast cancer: an update. J Clin Oncol 24:1940-1949
3. Fisher B, Saffer E, Rudock C et al (1989) Effect of local or systemic treatment prior to primary tumor removal on the production and response to a serum growth-stimulating factor in mice. Cancer Res 49:2002-2004
4. Fisher B, Brown A, Mamounas E et al (1997) Effect of preoperative chemotherapy on local-regional disease in women with operable breast cancer: findings from National Surgical Adjuvant Breast and Bowel Project B-18. J Clin Oncol 15:2483-2493
5. Mauri D, Pavlidis N, Ioannidis JP (2005) Neoadjuvant versus adjuvant systemic treatment in breast cancer: a meta-analysis. J Natl Cancer Inst 97:188-194
6. Berruti A, Brizzi MP, Generali D et al (2008) Presurgical systemic treatment of nonmetastatic breast cancer: facts and open questions. Oncologist 13:1137-1148
7. Prati R, Minami CA, Gornbein JA et al (2009) Accuracy of clinical evaluation of locally advanced breast cancer in patients receiving neoadjuvant chemotherapy. Cancer 115:1194-1202
8. Mann RM, Kuhl CK, Kinkel K, Boetes C (2008) Breast MRI: guidelines from the European Society of Breast Imaging. Eur Radiol 18:1307-1318
9. Tardivon AA, Ollivier L, El Khoury C, Thibault F (2006) Monitoring therapeutic efficacy in breast carcinomas. Eur Radiol 16:2549-2558
10. Sardanelli F, Boetes C, Borisch B et al (2010) Magnetic resonance imaging of the breast: recommendations from the EUSOMA working group. Eur J Cancer 46:1296-1316
11. Buchholz TA, Lehman CD, Harris JR et al (2008) Statement of the science concerning locoregional treatments after preoperative chemotherapy for breast cancer: a National Cancer Institute conference. J Clin Oncol 26:791-797
12. Vinnicombe SJ, MacVicar AD, Guy RL et al (1996) Primary breast cancer: mammographic changes after neoadjuvant chemotherapy, with pathologic correlation. Radiology 198:333–340
13. Moskovic EC, Mansi JL, King DM et al (1993) Mammography in the assessment of response to medical treatment of large primary breast cancer. Clin Radiol 47:339–344
14. Huber S, Wagner M, Zuna I et al (2000) Locally advanced breast carcinoma: evaluation of mammography in the prediction of residual disease after induction chemotherapy. Anticancer

Res 20:553–558
15. Helvie MA, Joynt LK, Cody RL et al (1996) Locally advanced breast carcinoma: accuracy of mammography vs clinical examination in the prediction of residual disease after chemotherapy. Radiology 198:327–332
16. Croshaw R, Shapiro-Wright H, Svensson E et al (2011) Accuracy of clinical examination, digital mammogram, ultrasound, and MRI in determining postneoadjuvant pathologic tumor response in operable breast cancer patients. Ann Surg Oncol 18:3160-3163. Epub Sep 27, 2011
17. Balu-Maestro C, Chapellier C, Bleuse A et al (2002) Imaging in evaluation of response to neoadjuvant breast cancer treatment benefits in MRI. Breast Cancer Res Treat 72:145–152
18. Schott ZF, Roubidoux MA, Helvie MA et al (2002) Clinical and radiological assessments to predict breast cancer pathologic complete response to neoadjuvant chemotherapy. Breast Cancer Res Treat 92:231–238
19. Roubidoux MA, Le Carpentier GL, Fowles JB et al (2005) Sonographic evaluation of early-stage breast cancers that undergo neoadjuvant chemotherapy. J Ultrasound Med 24:885–895
20. Rieber A, Brambs HJ, Gabelmann A et al (2002) Breast MRI for monitoring response of primary breast cancer to neo-adjuvant chemotherapy. Eur Radiol 7:1711–1719
21. Yuan Y, Chen XS, Liu SY, Shen KW (2010) Accuracy of MRI in prediction of pathologic complete remission in breast cancer after preoperative therapy: a meta-analysis. AJR 195(1):260-268
22. Montemurro F, Martincich L, De Rosa G et al (2005) Dynamic contrast-enhanced MRI and sonography in patients receiving primary chemotherapy for breast cancer. Eur Radiol 15:1224-1233
23. Thibault F, Nos C, Meunier M et al (2004) MRI for surgical planning in patients with breast cancer who undergo preoperative chemotherapy. Am J Roentgenol 183:1159–1168
24. Wasser K, Klein SK, Fink C et al (2003) Evaluation of neoadjuvant chemotherapeutic response of breast cancer using dynamic MRI with high temporal resolution. Eur Radiol 13:80–87
25. Loo CE, Straver ME, Rodenhuis S et al (2011) Magnetic resonance imaging response monitoring of breast cancer during neoadjuvant chemotherapy: relevance of breast cancer subtype. J Clin Oncol 29:660-666
26. Padhani AR, Liu G, Koh DM et al (2009) Diffusion-weighted magnetic resonance imaging as a cancer biomarker: consensus and recommendations. Neoplasia 11:102-125
27. Woodhams R, Kakita S, Hata H et al (2010) Identification of residual breast carcinoma following neoadjuvant chemotherapy: diffusion-weighted imaging—comparison with contrast-enhanced MR imaging and pathologic findings. Radiology 254:357-366
28. Partridge SC, Gibbs JE, Lu Y et al (2005) MRI measurements of breast tumor volume predict response to neoadjuvant chemotherapy and recurrence-free survival. AJR Am J Roentgenol 184:1774-1781
29. Martincich L, Montemurro F, De Rosa G et al (2004) Monitoring response to primary chemotherapy in breast cancer using dynamic contrast enhanced magnetic resonance imaging. Breast Cancer Res Treat 83:67-76
30. Cheung YC, Chen SC, Su MY et al (2003) Monitoring the size and response of locally advanced breast cancers to neoadjuvant chemotherapy (weekly paclitaxel and epirubicin) with serial enhanced MRI. Breast Cancer Res Treat 78:51–58
31. El Khoury C, Servois V, Thibault F et al (2005) MR quantification of the washout changes in breast tumors under preoperative chemotherapy: feasibility and preliminary results. Am J Roentgenol 184:1499–1504
32. Leach MO, Brindle KM, Evelhoch JL et al (2003) Assessment of antiangiogenic and antivascular therapeutics using MRI: recommendations for appropriate methodology for clinical trials. Br J Radiol 76 Spec No 1:S87-S91
33. Padhani AR, Hayes C, Assersohn L et al (2006) Prediction of clinicopathologic response of breast cancer to primary chemotherapy at contrast-enhanced MR imaging: initial clinical results. Radiology 239:361-374
34. Ah-See ML, Makris A, Taylor NJ et al (2008) Early changes in functional dynamic magnetic resonance imaging predict for pathologic response to neoadjuvant chemotherapy in primary breast cancer. Clin Cancer Res 14:6580-6589

35. Sardanelli F, Fausto A, Podo F (2008) MR spectroscopy of the breast. Radiol Med 113:56-64

36. Jagannathan NR, Kumar M, Seenu V et al (2001) Evaluation of total choline from in vivo volume localized proton MR spectroscopy and its response to neoadjuvant chemotherapy in locally advanced breast cancer. Br J Cancer 84:1016–1022

37. Tozaki M, Sakamoto M, Oyama Y et al (2010) Predicting pathological response to neoadjuvant chemotherapy in breast cancer with quantitative 1H MR spectroscopy using the external standard method. J Magn Reson Imaging 31:895-902

38. Meisamy S, Bolan PJ, Baker EH et al (2004) Neoadjuvant chemotherapy of locally advanced breast cancer: predicting response with in vivo (1) HMR spectroscopy-a pilot study at 4 T. Radiology 233:424–431

39. Hamstra DA, Rehemtulla A, Ross BD (2007) Diffusion magnetic resonance imaging: a biomarker for treatment response in oncology. J Clin Oncol 25:4104-4109

40. Park SH, Moon WK, Cho N et al (2010) Diffusion-weighted MR imaging: pretreatment prediction of response to neoadjuvant chemotherapy in patients with breast cancer. Radiology 257:56-63

41. Pickles MD, Gibbs P, Lowry M, Turnbull LW (2006) Diffusion changes precede size reduction in neoadjuvant treatment of breast cancer. Magn Reson Imaging 24:843-847

Lung Cancer

7

Massimo Bellomi, Tommaso De Pas, Adele Tessitore and Lorenzo Preda

7.1   Introduction

Lung cancer is the most frequent cancer-related cause of death [1] and the management of locally advanced non-small-cell lung cancer (NSCLC) remains a challenge. Both local relapses and distant metastases are frequent, with a 5-year survival of 3–17% for inoperable disease [2]. According to the data released by the IASLC Lung Cancer Staging Project in 2007, the 5-year survival rates for the new clinical stages were 50%, 47%, 36%, 26%, 19%, 7%, and 2% for IA, IB, IIA, IIB, IIIA, IIIB, and IV, respectively. Table 7.1 indicates the corresponding survival for their pathological counterparts [3].

Since the surgical resection of lung cancer offers the best chance of cure, accurate staging is important to determine which patients are candidates for surgery. In general, clinical stages I, II, and in some cases IIIA and exceptionally IIIB are considered as resectable disease, whereas more extensive disease, as seen in other cases of stage IIIA and in most cases of stage IIIB and IV, are usually treated with radiation therapy, chemotherapy, or a combination of the two [4]. In this review, we discuss patients with stage III disease in greater detail, because they are most likely to also be candidates for neoadjuvant treatment. Therefore, an accurate operative staging and the definition of response to preoperative chemo-radiotherapy is of great revelance.

M. Bellomi (✉)
Radiology Unit, European Institute of Oncology, Milan; Department of Medicine and Surgery, University of Milan, Milan, Italy

M. Aglietta, D. Regge (eds.), *Imaging Tumor Response to Therapy,* © Springer-Verlag Italia 2012   109

Table 7.1 5-year lung cancer survival in relation to pathological stage

Stage	pTNM subset	5-year survival
0	Carcinoma in situ	
IA	T1a/T1b, N0M0	73%
IB	T2aN0M0	58%
IIA	T1a/T1b, N1M0 T2aN1M0 T2b N0M0	46%
IIB	T2bN1M0 T3N0M0	36%
IIIA	T1/T2, N2M0 T3, N1/N2, M0 T4, N0/N1, M0	24%
IIIB	T4N2M0 Any T, N3, M0	9%
IV	Any T, any N, M1a/M1b	13%

7.2   Treatment Strategies for Patient with Clinical Stage III Disease

Stage III can be further divided in two subgroups. Stage IIIA comprises a heterogeneous group of patients with ipsilateral cancer, including T3 lesions with hilar lymphatic involvement (N1) and/or mediastinal ipsilateral involvement (N2); T4 lesions (invasion of the trachea, carina, heart, great vessels, vertebral body, esophagus, or mediastinum, one or more satellite tumor nodule (s) in the same lung but in a lobe other than the one involved by the primary mass) without or with hilar lymphatic involvement (N0, N1); and any tumor size with mediastinal lymphatic metastasis (N2) [3]. Mediastinal involvement (N2 disease) is associated with a 5-year survival of 25% or less. However, several studies have shown a significant clinical benefit of radical surgery in patients with a complete mediastinal response to induction therapy. For patients with low tumor burden, considered resectable at diagnosis, the aim of induction therapy is to optimize distant disease control by the administration of chemotherapy at the time of the lowest micrometastatic burden.

Stage IIIB includes patients with a primary tumor of any size and supraclavicular or contralateral mediastinal nodal metastases (T1–4, N3) as well as T4 lesions with ipsilateral mediastinal lymph node involvement (N2) [3]. Nowadays, this stage is an absolute contraindication to surgery and patients are usually treated with chemo-radiation therapy. However, in a phase II study in which stage IIIB patients underwent induction chemotherapy and radiotherapy followed by surgery, the Southwest Oncology Group reported results similar to those obtained in patients with N2 disease [4].

7.2.1   Neoadjuvant Chemotherapy

Neoadjuvant chemotherapy is usually proposed for patients with stage IIIA N2 disease, in order to reduce the tumor bulk, address micrometastatic disease [5], and improve clinical outcome. Induction chemotherapy regimens include platinum-based doublets administered for up to four cycles; the overall response rate is approximately 60%. Giving induction chemotherapy, pathological downstaging (pN0 - pN1) may be obtained in about 40 -60% of these cases, with 5-10% of pathological complete response. In terms of overall survival, randomized trials comparing neoadjuvant platinum-based regimens with surgery alone demonstrated a benefit for pharmacological treatment before surgery A meta-analysis of 988 patients from seven randomized trials confirmed the overall survival improvement in patients who underwent neoadjuvant chemotherapy (20%; p=0.02) compared with the observation group (14%) [6]. Furthermore, neoadjuvant chemotherapy is usually not associated with a higher surgical morbidity. Other candidates for neoadjuvant chemotherapy are non-N2 patients with locally advanced disease (T4), in order to reduce tumor size and facilitate surgical approaches.

7.2.2   Unresectable Locally Advanced Disease

Currently, chemo-radiotherapy is the standard of care for patients with stage IIIB disease and for those with unresectable stage IIIA tumors. Platinum-containing chemotherapy can be administered either before or together with chest radiotherapy. Meta-analyses comparing sequential versus concomitant chemotherapy highlighted the advantage of the latter regimen in terms of overall survival, while no differences were observed for progression-free survival or for the control of distant metastases [7]. The advantage in the control of loco-regional disease might reside in the radio-sensitizing effect of chemotherapy, which improves the efficacy of radiotherapy. The cost is the increase in toxicity, consisting mainly of severe acute esophagitis.

7.3   Monitoring the Response to Treatment by Uni- and Bi-dimensional Measurements

Conventionally, the response assessment criteria (WHO and RECIST) used in patients with locally advanced lung cancer are based, as in other solid tumors, on size measurements (see Chapter 2 for further details).

In lung cancer, multi-detector CT (MDCT) is the most frequently used imaging technique in the evaluation of both pulmonary and mediastinal disease. According to the RECIST criteria, CT scans should be performed with a contiguous slice thickness of ≤ 5 mm; with these parameters, a minimum of 10 mm is considered measurable at baseline. The lesions should be measured on

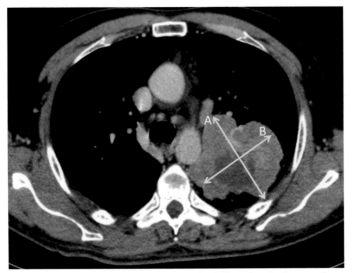

Fig. 7.1 A 61-year-old man with a poorly differentiated adenocarcinoma of the left lung. CT demonstrates a large, lobulated mass in the left upper lobe. The tumor was measured using the WHO ($A \times B$) and RECIST (A) criteria, where A represents the longest diameter of the lesion and B the longest perpendicular distance

axial images and always at the same window setting (Fig. 7.1). Size can be determined on the reconstructed images if isotropic imaging is performed. Large, non-nodal pulmonary lesions should be measured on the slice where the tumor diameter is the greatest. Lung or soft-tissue windows can be used according to RECIST to measure lung lesions, providing the same window setting is used throughout the studies. A soft-tissue window allows better differentiation of large lesions, i.e., involving the main bronchi, from distally located atelectasis of the lung parenchyma (Fig. 7.2).

Irregular or spiculated lesions are a common finding in the advanced stages of lung cancer and their measurement is particularly challenging. Optimal visualization of the spicules is achieved with the lung window setting, while these pathologic structures are less apparent with a soft-tissue setting. However, the latter window provides a more accurate visualization of the solid-tumor components [8] (Fig. 7.3). Unfortunately RECIST does not specify whether the measurements should include the entire length of the spicule or limited to the solid portion of the lesions.

Tumors situated in a previously irradiated area are usually not considered measurable, according to RECIST, unless disease progression can be clearly demonstrated [9]. Radiation-induced imaging changes are a common finding and they may severely limit the ability of CT to detect recurrence, especially in the initial 6 months after therapy [10]. Radiation pneumonitis is an acute or subacute inflammatory reaction of the lung parenchyma, usually confined to the field of irradiation and occurring within 1–6 months of treatment. The imaging

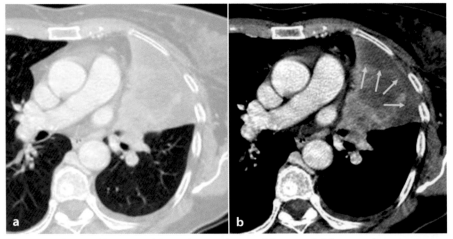

Fig. 7.2 A 56-year-old woman with an adenocarcinoma of the upper left lung causing complete at-electasis of the upper lobe. Same CT scan imaged with a lung setting (**a**) and a soft-tissue setting (**b**). In this case, the latter better differentiates between the lesion and the atelectatic lung parenchyma (*arrows*)

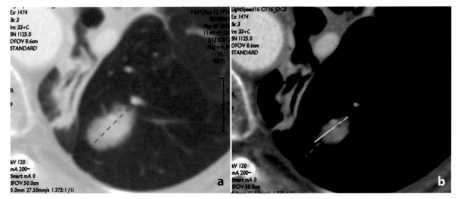

Fig. 7.3 a CT measurement of the maximum diameter of a lesion in the left lower lobe imaged with a lung setting. **b** In the same scan but imaged with a soft-tissue setting, the size of the lesion is greatly reduced

changes include diffuse consolidation, patchy consolidation associated with ground-glass opacities, which may be diffuse or patchy [11, 12]. Imaging findings may lag behind clinical symptoms, which usually consist of cough, fever, shortness of breath, and chest pain, by weeks to months (Fig. 7.4) [13].

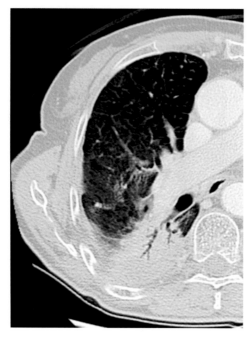

Fig. 7.4 Radiation pneumonitis in a 75-year-old woman treated with radiotherapy 5 months earlier for NSCLC in the right lower lobe. CT scan shows an area of consolidation with an air-bronchogram

Up to 10% of patients receiving radiotherapy develop radiation fibrosis, typically 6–24 months after treatment, as a consequence of radiation pneumonitis or airways injury [10]. The radiological pattern is characterized by consolidation, volume loss, traction bronchiectasis and bronchiolectasis, architectural distortion, and pleural thickening (Fig. 7.5a) [13]. The presence of these radiation-induced imaging changes, especially mass-like consolidations, may preclude the early detection of disease persistence or recurrence. In these cases, one must search for the following CT features of tumor recurrence: an increase in the size of the consolidation sometime after the initial decrease, the development of a soft-tissue mass or convexity along the lateral border of radiation fibrosis, and the filling of ectatic bronchi (Fig. 7.5b) [10].

Inter-observer agreement is considered acceptable when small, well-defined pulmonary nodules are measured. However, in clinical practice, in which large and irregular tumors are most often encountered, different studies have demonstrated the very high variability in lesion measurements by different readers [8, 11, 12]. Erasmus et al. [8] used RECIST to assess inter- and intra-observer variability in 40 patients with NSCLCs. In their study, disease progression was erroneously determined to have occurred in 30% and 9.5% of lesions measured by different observers or measured repeatedly by the same observers, respectively. In addition, it must be kept in mind that the WHO criteria and RECIST are based on the assumption that the tumor undergoes sym-

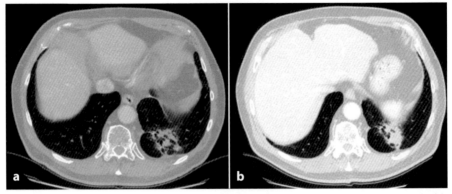

Fig. 7.5 An 80-year-old man with a squamocellular carcinoma of the left lower lobe treated with radiotherapy. **a** The CT scan obtained 7 months after the end of the treatment shows signs of post-radiation fibrosis with patchy consolidation and traction bronchiectasis. **b** The scan taken 5 months later shows the development of a soft-tissue mass along the lateral border of radiation fibrosis, with filling of the ectatic bronchi, suggestive of recurrence

metric changes and that size can be expressed by planar measurements. In actuality, however, different portions of the tumor may grow or respond to therapies at different rates. Therefore, to improve the assessment of change in tumor size there is a need for other, radically different approaches to measurement [14].

7.4   Measuring Tumor Volume

Today, MDCT technology allows large anatomic volumes to be examined with high resolution on all three planes of imaging (i.e., isotropic imaging) [15]. In the measurement of lung nodules, the specialized software used to estimate the growth rate of small lung nodules has been recently replaced by 3D methods [16-19], which yield more accurate and consistent tumor measurements as well as accurate determinations of temporal changes in a shorter interval [15, 16]. Zhao et al. [20] performed CT volumetry on scans of 15 patients with NSCLC, both before and after gefitinib treatment. They found that, compared to 1- and 2D techniques, the use of semi-automated algorithms to calculate tumor volume enabled the identification of 20–30% more patients with absolute changes. The same authors measured the reproducibility and repeatability of lung-cancer CT volume measurements by scanning patients twice on the same day [17]. They concluded that volume differences measured on the serial scans outside the range of -12.1–13.4% could be considered true changes in tumor volume [16, 17]. Bendsten et al. [21] showed that volumet-

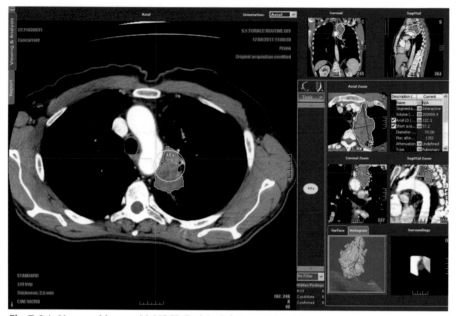

Fig. 7.6 A 61-year-old man with NSCLC of the left upper lobe. A 3D segmentation algorithm from a commercially available volume analysis software (LMS, Median Technologies, France) distinguishes the mass from the mediastinal structures, allowing CT volume measurement (expressed in mm^3) of the tumor

ric analysis is feasible with high accuracy and low variability also in the context of advanced NSCLC with complex lesions. In these cases, while the use of semi-automated segmentation is critical for the reduction of operator variability, manual refinement and segmentation are still necessary to properly separate the lesion boundary from adjacent normal structures (Fig. 7.6) [21]

The above-reported studies show that computer-assisted diagnosis may help to differentiate response patterns in patients categorized by RECIST as having stable disease [22]. However, volume measurements need to be standardized and made widely available before volumetric response criteria can be universally accepted and integrated in routine oncological practice. Furthermore, computer-assisted measurements may be challenging in the volume assessments of complex or cavitary masses, which are common findings in patients with advanced NSCLC. Technical advances, such as improved segmentation, are needed to overcome these challenges, which have become even greater with the advent of targeted therapies, as discussed below [22].

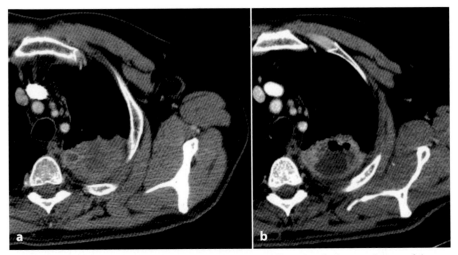

Fig 7.7 CT scans from a 61-year-old man with a poorly differentiated adenocarcinoma of the upper left lobe before (**a**) and after (**b**) two cycles of chemotherapy including a targeted-cytostatic agent. After treatment, there was no significant decrease in the size of the mass, but CT shows the appearance of necrosis and cavitation inside the lesion

7.5   Functional Imaging: Positron Emission Tomography

There is increasing awareness that the evaluation of treatment response based solely on tumor size measurement has important limitations, especially since the introduction of targeted agents, which frequently produce lesion cavitation [23] (Fig. 7.7). Accordingly, the emphasis has shifted to "functional" imaging techniques capable of depicting changes in cellular activities [22, 23].

The role of ^{18}F-FDG PET to assess treatment response in NSCLC has been extensively studied in the last decade [22]. In 2007, de Geus-Oei et al., [24] reviewed nine PET studies of patients with advanced NSCLC. They reported that a > 20% decrease in SUV after one cycle of chemotherapy was associated with a longer time to progression and that median overall survival was significantly longer in patients with stage IIIA-N2 disease who had a complete metabolic response. Similarly, Nahmias et al. [25] determined that the results of ^{18}F-FDG PET evaluations carried out 1 and 3 weeks after the beginning of chemotherapy in patients with advanced NSCLC were predictive of the response to treatment.

The role of ^{18}F-FDG PET in the evaluation of patients with NSCLC who underwent radiotherapy is also well established. A normal ^{18}F-FDG PET study in patients with radiation-induced imaging changes is highly predictive of a negative result [10]. Conversely, Patz et al. [26] demonstrated that patients with residual tumor or recurrence after radiotherapy had high SUV values.

They identified a cut-off value of 2.5 as the best threshold between normal and pathological findings. As a general rule, the presence of ^{18}F-FDG PET activity similar to that of pre-treatment levels, associated with worrisome CT findings, should be considered highly suspicious [10].

Disease restaging in patients with advanced, but potentially resectable NSCLC (stage IIIA-N2) treated with neoadjuvant chemotherapy is particularly challenging. Indeed, several studies have demonstrated that pathological downstaging or clearance of disease in the mediastinal lymph nodes is crucial for a favorable outcome. In 2010, Rebollo-Aguirre et al. [27] systematically reviewed all data from the literature on patients with NSCLC N2 that had been staged with ^{18}F-FDG PET. They found that the overall sensitivity and specificity of ^{18}F-FDG PET were 63.8% (95% CI, 53.3–73.7%) and 85.3% (95% CI, 80.4–89.4%) respectively. The authors concluded that, despite the better results of PET/CT compared to cross-sectional imaging alone (Fig. 7.8), the use of a non-invasive diagnostic approach is not recommended as the only reassessment tool for mediastinal lymph node evaluation; rather, an invasive technique, such as endoscopic ultrasound-guided aspiration biopsy or re-do mediastinoscopy, should be considered for restaging purposes [27].

PET tracers are becoming available to evaluate other specific biological characteristics of the tumors, besides glucose metabolism. Among these, ^{18}F-fluorothymidine (^{18}F-FLT) PET may have a role in evaluating the response to therapy in lung cancer, particularly when the treatment approach includes inhibitors of proliferative activity such as cyclin-dependent kinase inhibitors [22].

7.6   Functional Imaging with MRI and CT

Dynamic contrast-enhanced MRI (DCE-MRI) and CT-perfusion (CTp) are new, non-invasive and reproducible methods that allow the quantitative assessment of tumor vascularity in vivo (Fig. 7.9) [28-31]. DCE-MRI has attracted attention with respect to several aspects: as a potential biomarker of tumor phenotype, as a measure of response to therapy, and as a prognostic factor in different types of cancer, including NSCLC. Initially, it was used to evaluate pulmonary perfusion and to characterize pulmonary solitary nodules [32-36]. More recently, the value of DCE-MRI as a prognostic marker of treatment response has been studied [37, 38]. For example, Ohno et al. [38] evaluated 114 patients with lung cancer being treated with cisplatin and vincristine. They observed a significantly lower maximum relative enhancement ratio and a flatter slope of enhancement in the group of patients with a better prognosis; the mean survival period of patients with a slope of enhancement ≤ 0.08/s was significantly longer. These preliminary data are promising in terms of the use of DCE-MRI in the assessment of lung cancer response to chemotherapy and targeted therapy.

Diffusion weighted imaging (DW-MRI) is an alternative approach to DCE-MRI that in the future may have a significant role as an imaging marker (Fig. 7.10).

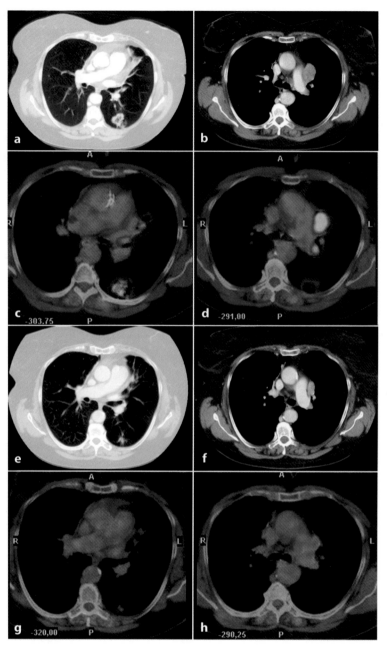

Fig. 7.8 A 63-year-old woman with a T2-N2 NSCLC in the left lower lobe. **a, b** Baseline CT shows a 3.2-cm pulmonary lesion and an enlarged subaortic node (station 5 according to the American Thoracic Society classification), **c, d** both of which showed FDG uptake at PET/CT. **e, f** After three cycles of chemotherapy, the mass as well as the node decreased significantly in size, but both were still evident at CT. **g, h** PET/CT shows the persistence of slight FDG uptake only in the subaortic node

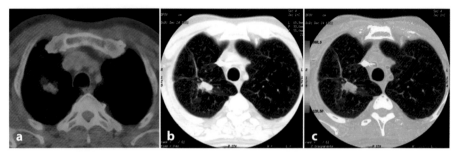

Fig. 7.9 A 56-year-old patient with a solid benign lesion localized in the right upper lung lobe. **a** CT scan documents a solid lesion with a non-calcific density. **b** A blood-flow color map shows the solid lesion as predominantly blue, indicating low flow levels. **c** On PET/CT, there is no significant FDG uptake

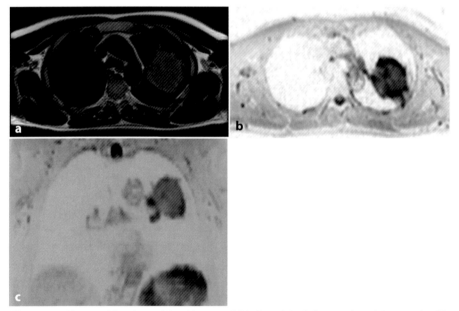

Fig. 7.10 A 50-year-old patient with a 64-mm solid lesion of the left upper lung lobe (poorly differentiated acinar-and-solid mixed adenocarcinoma). **a** T2 weighted MRI documents a solid lesion with pleural infiltration. **b** Diffusion-weighted axial image ($b = 1000$ s/mm^2) with gray-scale inversion: the lesion is a darker shade of gray than the suppressed background tissues, due to its high cellularity. **c** Coronal reconstruction of the diffusion-weighted image

Yabuuchi et al. [39] used DW-MRI to evaluate 28 stage IIIB and IV tumors before and after the first course of chemotherapy. The authors found a significant correlation between the change in the apparent diffusion coefficient (ADC, see Chapter 2) after the first course of chemotherapy and both final tumor size reduction and progression-free survival.

7.7   Conclusions

Data obtained from different functional techniques are increasingly being combined such that multifunctional evaluation is becoming an important approach to the biological investigation of cancer. Several studies evaluating relationships between perfusion parameters measured with TCp, such as blood flow, and glucose metabolism, as measured by ^{18}F-FDG PET, have been investigated in a large variety of tumors, including NSCLC [40]. Interestingly, a flow-metabolism mismatch has been determined in high-grade and larger, advanced tumors. Miles et al. [41] suggested that low vascularity with high glucose uptake represents an adequate tumor adaptation to hypoxic stress. This adaptative behavior was shown to be associated with poorer patient outcome [42]. Tumor heterogeneity is a second well-recognized feature related to adverse tumor biology and is of potential relevance in treatment response. Texture analysis using non-contrast-enhanced CT images is emerging as a novel approach to evaluate tumor heterogeneity, by quantifying local variations in image brightness within a pulmonary lesion [43]. A study by Ganeshan et al. [43] provided preliminary evidence for a relationship between texture and FDG uptake on PET and tumor stage, concluding that texture analysis warrants further investigations as a method of obtaining prognostic information for patients with NSCLC who are undergoing CT.

Despite their limitations, 1D measurements and changes in glucose metabolism still represent the mainstay in the evaluation of the response to therapy of advanced NSCLC. Today's technologies are expanding the potential of imaging markers, whose thorough validation will be needed before they can be employed to predict and evaluate response to treatment. At this point in time, the ability of multiparametric and multifunctional imaging to better reflect tumor heterogeneity and biological behavior is still speculative.

Clinical Case

A 75-year-old male, a previous smoker, with locally advanced non-small cell lung cancer (NSCLC) was treated with six cycles of induction chemotherapy containing cisplatin (CDDP) plus gemcitabine (GCB).

Baseline CT of the chest demonstrated a 3.4-cm mass in the left upper lobe (Fig. 7.11a) and a metastatic hilar adenopathy (station 10L according to the American Thoracic Society classification) not dissociable from the pulmonary artery (Fig. 7.11b). At pre-treatment PET/CT, both the primary lesion and the metastatic node showed intense FDG uptake (Fig. 7.11c, d). Clinical and imaging evaluation resulted in a pre-treatment staging of cT2–cN1.

CT evaluation at the end of systemic chemotherapy showed a decrease in the size of the pulmonary lesion and the hilar node; at the site of the primary tumor, a 1.8-cm spiculated mass was still evident, considered suspicious for residual disease (Fig. 7.12a,b).

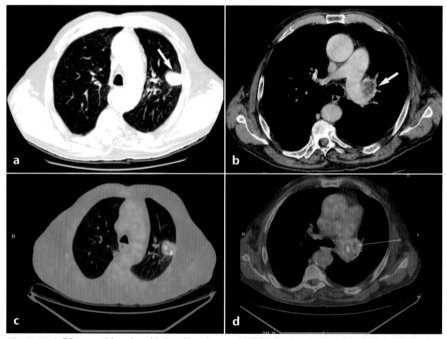

Fig. 7.11 A 75-year-old male with locally advanced NSCLC treated with six cycles of induction chemotherapy followed by surgery. Baseline CT examination demonstrates a 3.4-cm mass in the left upper lobe (*white arrow*) (**a**) and a metastatic hilar adenopathy with a 3.0-cm short axis (station 10L according to the ATS; *white arrow*) (**b**). **c, d** ¹⁸F-FDG PET/CT shows intense metabolic activitity of both the primary lesion and the metastatic node

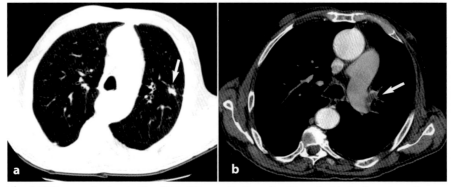

Fig. 7.12 Same patient as in Fig. 7.11. CT examination after the end of induction chemotherapy shows the persistence of a 1.8-cm spiculated lesion in the left upper lobe (*white arrow*) (**a**) and a 1.0-cm short axis hilar node (*white arrow*) (**b**), both considered suspicious for persistent disease

Post-treatment ^{18}F-FDG PET showed only a slight, not significant metabolic activity at the level of both the pulmonary lesion and the hilum (not shown). A left pneumonectomy with radical lymphoadenectomy was performed. Pathological response was a complete tumor response: ypT0 ypN0. No disease recurrence was reported during subsequent follow up.

References

1. http://seer.cancer.gov
2. Roger S, Mayer M, Kann R et al (2009) Neoadjuvant chemotherapy and radiotherapy followed by surgery in selected patients with stage IIIB non-small-cell lung cancer: a multicentre phase II trial. Lancet Oncol 10:785-93
3. Goldstraw P, Crowley J, Chansky K et al; International Association for the Study of Lung Cancer International Staging Committee; Participating Institutions (2007) The IASLC Lung Cancer Staging Project: proposals for the revision of the TNM stage groupings in the forthcoming (seventh) edition of the TNM Classification of malignant tumours. J Thorac Oncol 2(8):706-14. Erratum in: J Thorac Oncol 2(10):985
4. Rusch VW, Albain KS, Crowley JJ et al (1993) Surgical resection of stage IIIA and stage IIIB non-small-cell lung cancer after concurrent induction chemoradiotherapy. A Southwest Oncology Group trial. J Thorac Cardiovasc Surg 105:97-104
5. De Leyn P, Lardonois D, van Schil P et al (2007) ESTS guidelines for preoperative lymphnode staging for NSCLC. Eur J Cardiothorac Surgery 32:1-8
6. Robinson LA, Wagner H Jr, Ruckdeschelo JC (2003) Treatment of stage IIIA non-small cell lung cancer. Chest 123:202-220
7. Burdett S, Stewart LA, Rydzewska L (2006) A systematic review and meta-analysis of the literature: chemotherapy and surgery versus surgery alone in non-small cell lung cancer. J Thorac Oncol 1:611-621
8. Erasmus JJ, Gladish GW, Broemeling L et al (2003) Interobserver and intraobserver variability in measurement of non-small-cell carcinoma lung lesions: implications for assessment of tumor response. J Clin Oncol 21:2574-82

9. Koenig TR, Munden RF, Erasmus JJ et al (2002) Radiation injury of the lung after three-dimensional conformal radiation therapy. AJR Am J Roentgenol 178:1383-8

10. Eradat J, Abtin F, Gutierrez A, Suh R (2011) Evaluation of treatment response after nonoperative therapy for early-stage non-small cell lung carcinoma. Cancer J 17:38-48

11. Wormanns D, Diederich S, Lentschig MG et al (2000) Spiral CT of pulmonary nodules: interobserver variation in assessment of lesion size. Eur Radiol 10:710-3

12. Hopper KD, Kasales CJ, Van Slyke MA et al (1996) Analysis of interobserver and intraobserver variability in CT tumor measurements. AJR Am J Roentgenol 167:851-4

13. Park KJ, Chung JY, Chun MS, Suh JH (2000) Radiation-induced lung disease and the impact of radiation methods on imaging features. Radiographics 20:83-98

14. Gavrielides MA, Kinnard LM, Myers KJ, Petrick N (2009) Noncalcified lung nodules: volumetric assessment with thoracic CT. Radiology 251:26-37

15. Zhao B, Schwartz LH, Moskowitz CS et al (2005) Pulmonary metastases: effect of CT section thickness on measurement -initial experience. Radiology 234:934-9

16. Rampinelli C, De Fiori E, Raimondi S et al (2009) In vivo repeatability of automated volume calculations of small pulmonary nodules with CT. AJR Am J Roentgenol 192:1657-61

17. Zhao B, James LP, Moskowitz CS et al (2009) Evaluating variability in tumor measurements from same-day repeat CT scans of patients with non-small cell lung cancer. Radiology 252:263-72

18. Yankelevitz DF, Reeves AP, Kostis WJ et al (2000) Small pulmonary nodules: volumetrically determined growth rates based on CT evaluation. Radiology 217:251-6

19. Kostis WJ, Yankelevitz DF, Reeves AP et al (2004) Small pulmonary nodules: reproducibility of three-dimensional volumetric measurement and estimation of time to follow-up CT. Radiology 231:446-52

20. Zhao B, Schwartz LH, Moskowitz CS et al (2006) Lung cancer: computerized quantification of tumor response -initial results. Radiology 241:892-8

21. Bendtsen C, Kietzmann M, Korn R et al (2011) X-ray computed tomography: semiautomated volumetric analysis of late-stage lung tumors as a basis for response assessments. Int J Biomed Imaging 2011:361589. Epub 2011 May 24

22. Nishino M, Jackman DM, Hatabu H et al (2011) Imaging of lung cancer in the era of molecular medicine. Acad Radiol 18:424-36

23. Padhani AR, Miles KA (2010) Multiparametric imaging of tumor response to therapy. Radiology 256:348-64

24. de Geus-Oei LF, van der Heijden HF, Corstens FH, Oyen WJ (2007) Predictive and prognostic value of FDG-PET in nonsmall-cell lung cancer: a systematic review. Cancer 110:1654-64

25. Nahmias C, Hanna WT, Wahl LM et al (2007) Time course of early response to chemotherapy in non-small cell lung cancer patients with 18F-FDG PET/CT. J Nucl Med 48:744-51

26. Patz EF Jr, Lowe VJ, Hoffman JM et al (1994) Persistent or recurrent bronchogenic carcinoma: detection with PET and 2-F-18.-2-deoxy-D-glucose. Radiology 191:379-82

27. Rebollo-Aguirre AC, Ramos-Font C, Villegas Portero R et al (2010) Is FDG-PET suitable for evaluating neoadjuvant therapy in non-small cell lung cancer? Evidence with systematic review of the literature. J Surg Oncol 101:486-94

28. Lee TY, Purdie TG, Stewart E (2003) CT imaging of angiogenesis. J Nucl Med 47:171-187

29. Petralia G, Bonello L, Viotti S et al (2010) CT perfusion in oncology: how to do it. Cancer Imaging 10:8-19

30. Padhani AR (2000) Dynamic contrast-enhanced MR imaging. Cancer Imaging 1:52-63

31. Hylton N (2006) Dynamic contrast-enhanced magnetic resonance imaging as an imaging biomarker. J Clin Oncol 24:3293-8

32. Hatabu H, Gaa J, Kim D et al (1996) Pulmonary perfusion: qualitative assessment with dynamic contrast-enhanced MRI using ultra-short TE and inversion recovery turbo FLASH. Magn Reson Med 36:503-8

33. Ohno Y, Hatabu H, Takenaka D et al (2002) Solitary pulmonary nodules: potential role of dynamic MR imaging in management initial experience. Radiology 224:503-11

34. Schaefer JF, Vollmar J, Schick F et al (2004) Solitary pulmonary nodules: dynamic contrast-enhanced MR imaging—perfusion differences in malignant and benign lesions. Radiology 232:544-53

35. Donmez FY, Yekeler E, Saeidi V et al (2007) Dynamic contrast enhancement patterns of solitary pulmonary nodules on 3D gradient-recalled echo MRI. AJR Am J Roentgenol 189:1380-1386

36. Zou Y, Zhang M, Wang Q et al (2008) Quantitative investigation of solitary pulmonary nodules: dynamic contrast-enhanced MRI and histopathologic analysis. AJR Am J Roentgenol 191:252-9

37. Fujimoto K, Abe T, Müller NL et al (2003) Small peripheral pulmonary carcinomas evaluated with dynamic MR imaging: correlation with tumor vascularity and prognosis. Radiology 227:786-93. Epub 2003 Apr 24

38. Ohno Y, Nogami M, Higashino T et al (2005) Prognostic value of dynamic MR imaging for non-small-cell lung cancer patients after chemoradiotherapy. J Magn Reson Imaging 21:775-783

39. Yabuuchi H, Hatakenaka M, Takayama K et al (2011) Non-small cell lung cancer: detection of early response to chemotherapy by using contrast-enhanced dynamic and diffusion-weighted MR imaging. Radiology 2011 Epub ahead of print

40. Miles KA, Griffiths MR, Keith CJ (2006) Blood flow-metabolic relationships are dependent on tumour size in non-small cell lung cancer: a study using quantitative contrast-enhanced computer tomography and positron emission tomography. Eur J Nucl Med Mol Imaging 33:22-8. Epub 2005 Sep 23

41. Miles KA, Williams RE (2008) Warburg revisited: imaging tumour blood flow and metabolism. Cancer Imaging 8:81-6

42. Mankoff DA, Dunnwald LK, Partridge SC, Specht JM (2009) Blood flow-metabolism mismatch: good for the tumor, bad for the patient. Clin Cancer Res 15:5294-6. Epub 2009 Aug 25

43. Ganeshan B, Abaleke S, Young RC et al (2010)Texture analysis of non-small cell lung cancer on unenhanced computed tomography: initial evidence for a relationship with tumour glucose metabolism and stage. Cancer Imaging 10:137-43

Pancreatic Cancer

8

Marcello Orsi, Claudio Losio, Michele Reni, Nadia Di Muzio,
Francesco De Cobelli and Alessandro Del Maschio

8.1 Therapeutic Strategies in Non-resectable Pancreatic Cancer

8.1.1 Chemotherapy

While pancreatic cancer has an inherited or rapidly acquired chemoresistance, a meta-analysis of data from published clinical trials reported a significant improvement in overall survival (OS) among patients receiving chemotherapy [1]. Nowadays, gemcitabine is widely accepted as the standard first-line therapy and as the reference treatment arm for clinical trials in this patient population [2, 3]. However, its anti-tumoral activity is disappointing because the response rate is around 10%, median survival about 6 months, and 1-year OS around 20%.

During the last 15 years, several combination chemotherapy regimens and target therapies have been compared to single-agent gemcitabine in phase III trials but all of them failed to significantly improve OS. In a randomized phase III trial, a PEFG regimen consisting of cisplatin, epirubicin, 5-fluorouracil (5-FU), and gemcitabine was shown to be significantly superior to gemcitabine in terms of progression-free survival (PFS) (hazards ratio (HR) 0.51; range 0.33–0.78), OS (HR 0.65; range 0.43–0.99), response rate, and clinical benefit, without impairing quality of life [4]. The regimen has been subsequently modified by the inclusion of oral capecitabine instead of 5-FU. This PEXG regimen reproduced the previously reported OS figures, with > 40% of patients alive at 1-year, and reduced the inconvenience associated with the need to use portable pumps, as well as complications of indwelling catheter

M. Orsi (✉)
Department of Radiology, San Raffaele Hospital,
Milan, Italy

infections, rupture, and thrombotic events, all of which were related to the delivery of 5-FU by continuous infusion [5].

Interestingly, other phase III trials suggested that drug combinations consisting of more than two agents could improve OS when compared to gemcitabine [6]. In particular, compared with gemcitabine, the combination of 5-FU, leucovorin, irinotecan, and oxaliplatin improved PFS (6.4 vs. 3.3 months; $p < 0.0001$) and OS (11.1 vs. 6.8 months; 1-year OS 48.4 vs. 20.6% $p < 0.0001$) in patients with metastatic disease but normal bilirubin and good performance status. The data from this phase III trial are difficult to interpret. Moreover, a generalization of the results should be made with caution as attention must be paid to the selection of the enrolled patients, on the basis of the better than expected standard arm outcome, and to the remarkable grade 3–4 toxicity, which is barely acceptable in the context of palliative therapy (neutropenia 46%, thrombocytopenia 9%, anemia 8%, fatigue 23%, vomiting 15%, diarrhea 13%, peripheral neuropathy 9%). Yet, taken together, these findings endorse the rationale for further exploring the use of more than two drugs as upfront treatment in pancreatic adenocarcinoma.

In the metastatic setting, palliation and the prolongation of survival are the main goals. The demonstration and quantification of tumor shrinkage are, however, relevant and open the way to the use of the most effective drug combinations in the neoadjuvant setting in locally advanced disease.

8.1.2   Radiotherapy

The role of radiotherapy for local control in patients with pancreatic cancer is controversial because of the premise that patients die as a result of distant metastases [7]. Radiotherapy alone demonstrated worse median survival than radiochemotherapy in the Mayo Clinic study (6 vs. 10 months) [8]. These results were confirmed by a GITSG (Gastro Intestinal Tumor Study Group) report [9]; thus, for the majority of subsequent studies radiotherapy is to be understood as radiochemotherapy.

Radiotherapy can be used in the adjuvant setting, after tumor resection, to reduce loco-regional relapses. The European Organization for Research and Treatment of Cancer (EORTC) [10] conducted a randomized study (EORTC 40891) in patients with resectable pancreatic or periampullary cancer, based on radiochemotherapy vs. observation. The adjuvant treatment failed to demonstrate a significantly better 2-year PFS or OS. The criticisms of this study are: only a few of the patients had pancreatic cancer; they did not receive maintenance therapy; and positive and negative margins, without stratification, were included. In addition, quality assurance of the radiotherapy in this trial was missing. The European Study Group for Pancreatic Cancer, (ESPAC-1 trial) [11] conducted the largest phase III study, between 1999 and 2000. The authors concluded that chemotherapy was of benefit, while chemoradiotherapy was detrimental. The trial was criticized because of the suboptimal dose of radiotherapy, the use of a split-course technique, and the fact that 5-FU was given as a bolus injection, known to be inferior to prolonged intravenous infusion schedules. The RTOG 97-04 study [12] used higher doses (50.4 Gy) of irradiation, comparing two different chemotherapy regimens: 5-FU in continuous infusion vs. 5-FU plus gemcitabine pre- and post-chemoradiation. All patients were treated with modern radiotherapy techniques, and prospective quality assurance was requested. Patients in the gemcitabine arm had better median OS for pancreatic-head tumors (20.6 vs. 16.9 months, $p = 0.033$), with a higher hematological G4 toxicity, but without a difference in the rate of febrile neutropenia. This study changed the standard adjuvant therapy for the NCI and NCCN. The superior quality and technique of chemoradiotherapy may explain this difference in the results, and it can be hypothesized that effective radiotherapy enhanced treatment benefits [13].

Conflicting conclusions arose from two of the last meta-analyses published. In the Khanna report [14], a relative weight was taken into account and an absolute gain in survival of 12% was calculated from adjuvant chemoradiotherapy after 2 years ($p= 0.011$, 95% CI, 3–21%), based on five randomized trials comparing surgery with chemoradiotherapy. Stocken [15] concluded that adjuvant chemoradiation is more effective than chemotherapy only after R1-resections, with a reduction of the HR of 28% (SD 19).The value of adjuvant radiochemotherapy is currently controversial, with different interpretations on either side of the Atlantic. Chemoradiotherapy represents the standard of care in North America, while in Europe adjuvant chemotherapy alone is often indicated after R0-resection, and chemoradiation after R1-resection. The abovementioned studies represent the basis for neoadiuvant strategies that rely on a combination of chemo- and radiotherapy.

The neoadjuvant radiochemotherapy concept has the same rationale as in other tumor localizations: any partial response to treatment reduces the tumor volume, potentially increasing the likelihood of a negative margin at surgery. Multimodality therapy is expected to be better tolerated prior to, rather than after a radical pancreaticoduodenectomy. Thus, neoadjuvant chemoradiotherapy should be considered for patients with borderline resectable disease, as determined through a complete clinical staging. No prospective phase III randomized study has been published regarding neoadjuvant radiochemotherapy. A meta-analysis of the neoadjuvant treatments (94% chemoradiotherapy and 6% chemotherapy only), involving more than 4000 patients, demonstrated that patients with non-resectable disease treated with neoadjuvant therapies can achieve a survival rate comparable to that of patients with initially resectable tumor (median OS 20.5 vs. 23.3 months) [16]. Nonetheless, no conclusions can be reached prior to the release of the results of the ongoing first randomized multicenter study of the Interdisciplinary Working Group Gastrointestinal Tumours [17]. Neoadjuvant therapy is expected to prolong survival by achieving higher rates of curative resections (R0) and ypN0 tumors, and to increase local tumor control. It has been suggested that patients with locally advanced, unresectable tumors could, in 20% of cases, reach tumor resectability after neoadjuvant chemoradiation. Finally, patients with "borderline resectable" disease are more likely to have R1- or R2-resections, and hence a neoadjuvant strategy could be employed to increase the prospect of an R0-resection.

At the time of diagnosis, locally advanced pancreatic cancer is seen in one third of patients, that is those with genuinely unresectable disease in the absence of distant metastases. The optimal treatment in these cases is currently under debate; the chance for cure is low with radiation alone. The GITSG study [9] of patients with unresectable pancreatic cancer randomized them in three arms: split-course radiotherapy to a total dose of 40 Gy with a concomitant bolus of 5-FU vs. split-course radiotherapy to a total dose of 60 Gy with a concomitant bolus of 5-FU vs. radiotherapy to a total dose of 60 Gy alone. A prolonged median survival (42.2 vs. 40.3 vs. 22.9 weeks) was shown in both concomitant chemotherapy arms. This trial also raised the possibility that, with chemotherapy, a higher dose of radiation is perhaps not necessary, as the 1-year survival rates were similar in the 60-Gy and 40-Gy arms. However, a recent phase III trial reported inferior results with combined treatment [18]. The radiation dose used in that study was suboptimal, only 40 Gy. The radiation techniques were also outdated in two 1980s studies, because most patients were treated with parallel as opposed to anterior and posterior portals, associated with higher rates of toxicity, and CT-based imaging was not required for treatment planning, which could have resulted in significant geographical misses. It is obvious that the meta-analysis including these reports did not provide a definitive answer [1]. The ECOG 4201 study examined modern radiotherapy techniques [19] and found a better OS in combined modality treatment: median OS 11 vs. 9.2 months, $p = 0.034$; 50 vs. 32% at 12 months, 29 vs. 11% at 18 months, and 12 vs. 4% at 24 months. Combinations of radiochemotherapy and neoadjuvant or adjuvant chemotherapy yielded a median OS of 13–15 months, but this approach is currently under investigation in the LAP07 trial [20]. Considering that in the majority of patients with locally advanced disease recurrence involves distant sites, the concept of induction chemotherapy was developed to improve the prognosis in this group. This strategy could allow the selection of patients who will benefit most from radiotherapy. Thus, patients who develop distant metastases during induction chemotherapy continue with chemotherapy alone. In a recently published non-randomized series [21], patients were treated with gemcitabine-based chemotherapy for 3 months and those with stable disease were treated with chemoradiation or chemotherapy alone. The median survival time of patients who underwent chemoradiation was significantly longer (15 vs. 11.7 months). This result is probably due to the stable disease obtained with induction chemotherapy. These data are promising but they must be confirmed in a well-designed study.

8.2   Conventional Imaging and Serum Markers to Monitor and Predict Response to Tumor Treatment

Locally advanced pancreatic cancer, in which the tumor involves the celiac axis or superior mesenteric vessels but has not metastasized, is by definition unresectable and represents about 25% of pancreatic cancer cases at presentation. For these patients, the goal of treatment is to increase survival, relieve symptoms and, in some cases, to downstage cancer to the point that the patient may undergo radical surgery. In this scenario, the goal of imaging techniques is the early evaluation of tumor response to anticancer treatment, mainly to spare patients ineffective therapies with systemic toxic effects.

The assessment of tumor response in locally advanced pancreatic cancer is traditionally performed by a combination of CT parameters and by measuring the serum values of tumor markers [2].

8.2.1   Computed Tomography

Multidetector computed tomography (MDCT) is the reference technique not only for staging but also for response evaluation, due to its high spatial resolution, availability, and short acquisition time.

According to the RECIST criteria, response to treatment of locally advanced pancreatic carcinoma can be assessed by MDCT by monitoring the change in the lesion's largest diameter. However, CT measurements with RECIST have limitations. First, pancreatic tumors often show poorly defined margins and infiltrative growth and are sometimes not well-distinguishable from surrounding fibrosis or a desmoplastic reaction; accordingly, measurements are not reliable [22]. A recent study emphasized that pancreatic tumors are not spherical in shape and, since RECIST criteria are based on the assumption that tumors are spherical objects, a 1D evaluation of pancreatic cancer treatment response may not be accurate [23]. Another limitation of MDCT and of other conventional radiographic methods is that tumor shrinkage usually becomes evident months after the beginning of treatment; in pancreatic cancer, which has an extremely poor prognosis, this is an important bias. The new anticancer agents, with targeted mechanisms of action and subsequent cytostatic rather than cytotoxic effects will probably further underline the inherent limitation of morpho-dimensional criteria [24].

8.2.2   Tumor Markers

A wide range of serum proteins has been evaluated in the search for biomarkers specific to pancreatic cancer. The pancreatic tumor marker carbohydrate antigen (CA) 19-9 has abnormal values in > 80% of patients with advanced pancreatic carcinoma and is routinely measured in serum to monitor the course of disease, both on and off treatment. Changes in serum CA 19-9 concentration during treatment have been proposed as a parameter of efficacy. Measuring CA 19-9 is faster, cheaper, and easier to perform than the evaluation of target lesions on conventional imaging. Furthermore, variations in CA 19-9 concentration during chemotherapy might serve not only as a prognostic factor but also as an early marker of response [25].

Unfortunately, according to a recent trial based on prospectively collected data from a large cohort of patients, an early decrease in CA 19-9 concentration is not associated with lengthened survival [26]. Furthermore, in that study there was no concordance between imaging response and tumor-marker response, because almost half of the patients with disease progression, as evidenced on CT, conversely showed a $\geq 50\%$ decrease in CA 19-9 concentration. These findings suggest that therapeutic decisions cannot be reliably made on the basis of early CA 19-9 kinetics [26].

Other proteins have been evaluated as serum markers of pancreatic cancer. The first biomarker used for diagnostic purposes was carcinoembryonic antigen (CEA). Nowadays CEA is also measured to evaluate tumor response; however, with a sensitivity of just 25–56% it is of little value in many patients.

Recently, several studies have proposed the use of panels of biomarkers in diagnosing and monitoring pancreatic tumor, but their performances in terms of sensitivity and specificity do not differ from that of single serum markers [27].

8.3   New Approaches to Evaluate and Predict Tumor Response to Treatment

Over the years, imaging has evolved from a simple tool capable of yielding only morphological information to a source of advanced and complex morpho-functional data. Multiple parameters relating to tumor vitality, neoangiogenesis, and tissue texture can now be explored by means of molecular imaging and/or new MRI sequences. Furthermore, specialized software generates reproducible semi-quantitative and quantitative measures. Operator time may be shortened due to the semi-automatic or fully automatic capabilities of these new approaches. As reported above, pancreatic cancer is usually difficult to outline, especially after therapy, such that monitoring of these patients will no doubt improve as experience with the use of these advanced imaging techniques grows.

8.3.1   Positron Emission Tomography

^{18}F-FDG PET is now widely used to monitor response to treatment in sugar-avid cancers. Some recent studies demonstrated that early changes in FDG uptake often predict clinical outcome according to the following rule: the greater the decrease in post-therapy uptake, the better the response.

In their study of a small series of patients undergoing neoadjuvant chemotherapy, Choi et al. [28] showed that ^{18}F-FDG PET responders have a higher mean survival than non-responders (23.2 vs. 11.3 months). Further studies will be required to determine whether a change in SUV values, or a numerical cut-off, can be identified that correlates with clinical prognostic factors such as survival, thus recommending its use for initial (and subsequent) treatment assessment. Currently, a significant role for ^{18}F-FDG PET alone in monitoring the treatment of locally advanced pancreatic cancer has yet to be demonstrated.

Moreover, PET imaging has important limitations in evaluating the pancreas. Inflammatory tissue may yield a false-positive result, while chronic pancreatitis, cystadenoma, retroperitoneal fibrosis, and lymphocyte infiltration are other common causes of false findings. Treatment-induced changes following either radiotherapy or chemotherapy, may also cause false-positive results. Conversely, since FDG uptake is related to tumor grade, PET findings may be falsely negative in low-grade tumors. The degree of FDG uptake is also influenced by diabetes mellitus, which is a common sequela of pancreatic malignancy. Therefore, negative PET results in patients with elevated plasma glucose should be interpreted with caution.

8.3.2 Perfusion Imaging

Perfusion imaging can measure quantitative parameters that are related to tumor vascularization and can be performed with either CT or MRI. With both techniques, several images are acquired in the same region of the body at constant time intervals after intravenous contrast medium administration. The high temporal resolution scan is processed by means of specialized software that extracts different parameters reflecting tumoral neoangiogenesis. The most relevant is K^{trans}, which represents the volume transfer constant between blood plasma and the extracellular-extravascular space. A response to anti-cancer treatment usually brings about a reduction in K^{trans}, reflecting a reduction in vessel number and permeability; this event occurs more typically in hypervascular tumors and after the administration of antiangiogenic drugs. Pancreatic cancer is usually hypovascular and therefore should not be an ideal candidate for perfusion imaging. However, Park et al. [29], using a 64-row CT scanner, were able to show that pre-treatment K^{trans} can predict response to treatment. Patients with a higher K^{trans} value at baseline responded better to chemoradiotherapy than patients with tumors with low pre-treatment values. These results may be due to the better delivery of chemotherapeutic agent to the tumor bed, which also enhances its radiosensitivity.

In MRI performed after the administration of a novel antiangiogenic drug, a significant reduction was noted in almost all perfusion parameters, including K^{trans}. This finding correlated with a decrease in tumor marker levels before a reduction in tumor size was seen on CT [30].

Perfusion techniques still need to be fully evaluated and have some limitations. The radiation dose required for perfusion CT is very high, while MRI suffers from motion artifacts. Furthermore, the post-processing results may be affected by exam technique, equipment, and mathematical modeling and therefore might not always be entirely reliable and reproducible.

8.3.3 Diffusion-Weighted Imaging

Previously, DW-MRI was employed to enhance the detection of pancreatic lesions and in their differential diagnosis [31]. However, Niwa et al. [32] recently evaluated DW-MRI as a possible surrogate marker to predict response to chemotherapy in patients with advanced pancreatic adenocarcinoma. Apparent diffusion coefficient (ADC) values were measured at middle and high b-values before chemotherapy in 63 patients, avoiding areas of necrosis while tracing the region of interest (ROI) to avoid measurement errors. The study found that the rate of tumor progression was significantly higher in patients with a lower high b-value ADC than in those with a higher ADC value.

Several authors have investigated the role of quantitative DWI in evaluating the effects of chemotherapy on solid tumors, particularly in the neoadjuvant setting (breast and rectal cancer). The results suggested that when a chemotherapeutic regimen is effective, then shortly after the beginning of therapy there is an increase in mean ADC values, reflecting cell blebbing and lysis, that generally precedes the decrease in contrast enhancement and volume. Unfortunately, no studies have yet reported the use of DWI in monitoring the response to treatment of locally advanced pancreatic cancer.

We recently presented the results of a study of 15 patients with stages III and IV pancreatic adenocarcinoma who were evaluated before and during the administration of a multidrug gemcitabine-based regimen. All patients underwent DW-MRI before and during treatment [33]. The scanning protocol included high-resolution T2 turbo-spin-echo sequences (to depict morphology), followed by a single-shot echo planar DWI sequence, at baseline and 2 weeks after every cycle, for a period of 2 months. Tumor mean areas and ADC values were calculated by tracing tumoral ROIs on T2 images. ADC maps obtained at the different steps of imaging were compared. Response was also evaluated at MDCT, on the basis of RECIST criteria, and according to CA 19-9 levels at 2–3 months.

Twelve of the 15 patients showed a significant increase in tumor ADC after 1 month of therapy compared to baseline (1.74 ± 0.26 vs. $1.46 \pm 0.24 \times 10^{-3}$ mm^2/s; $p = 0.001$). This was assumed to be related to drug-induced edema and necrosis, and the patients were therefore considered to be responders. Within the same time interval, tumor shrinkage was not yet appreciable. Conversely, in non-responsive patients (3/15), there was no significant increase in the ADC.

These preliminary results suggest the ability of DWI to accurately assess the early modifications of neoplastic tissue that are coherent with a favorable response to treatment and that these changes anticipate those of both morphological imaging and serum biomarkers. An increased ADC may reflect a higher degree of freedom of water molecules, owing to the loss of membrane integrity or to an increase in total extracellular fluid that, in turn, may correspond to a reduction in the overall number of tumor cells or in their size. A later decrease of ADC values was observed in all patients and could be explained by two opposite phenomena: the onset of fibrosis in responders and tumor growth in non-responders. However, when quantitative DWI becomes ineffective, traditional criteria (tumor size on CT and CA 19-9) regain their value.

Our experience points to the potential of DWI as a useful tool for monitoring the early effects of chemotherapeutic drugs in patients with pancreatic adenocarcinoma, by predicting response within the month following the beginning of treatment, thus overcoming the limitations of conventional CT and of serum biomarkers. To confirm these findings will require a larger number of patients and a longer follow-up. Such studies will also determine whether there is a correlation with more significant clinical endpoints.

Clinical Case

A 70-year-old man with a 3-month history of abdominal pain and weight loss was admitted to our hospital. Abnormal blood tests included mild elevation of total bilirubin (1.37 mg/dL) and glucose (179 mg/dL) and severe elevation of alkaline phosphatase (341 U/L) and γ-glutamyl transpeptidase (953 U/L). Abdominal ultrasound revealed a hypoechoic, ill-defined pancreatic mass at the level of the uncinate process, raising suspicion of primary cancer (Fig. 8.1). Very high serum CA 19.9 levels (567 IU/mL) were measured as well.

A pathological diagnosis of pancreatic adenocarcinoma was obtained by means of endoscopic-ultrasound-guided fine-needle aspiration. Contrast-enhanced MDCT, performed 2 days later, confirmed the diagnosis of a pancreatic primary (longest diameter: 30 mm) with involvement of the superior mesenteric vessels and no distant metastasis (stage III) (Fig. 8.2).

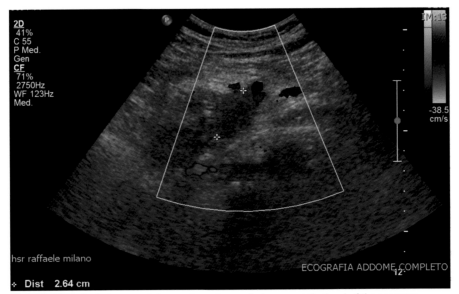

Fig. 8.1 Abdominal ultrasound shows a large hypoechoic mass at the head of the pancreas

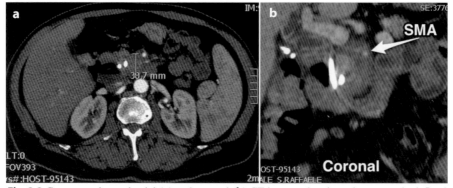

Fig. 8.2 Contrast-enhanced axial (**a**) and coronal (**b**) CT images showing a large, poorly defined 3-cm mass in the pancreatic head encasing the superior mesenteric artery (*white arrow*). At fine-needle biopsy, the lesion was diagnosed as adenocarcinoma

A neoadjuvant 4-drug chemotherapy regimen with gemcitabine, docetaxel, cisplatin, and capecitabin was initiated, with the cycles repeated every 28 days for a total of six courses. MRI scans with T2 turbo-spin-echo sequences followed by diffusion-weighted echo-planar imaging (b-values of 0 and 600 s/mm^2) were performed at baseline (Fig. 8.3) and every 2 weeks for the first 2 months of treatment for a total of five examinations. ADC maps were obtained from the diffusion-weighted images using dedicated software. The ADC was then estimated by tracing a ROI on the tumor boundary. A significant increase, from 1.40 to 1.79 × 10^{-3} mm^2/s (28%), in the ADC compared to the pre-treatment value was determined at the second MRI examination, only 1 month after the start of therapy and before any appreciable modification in tumor size and morphology as seen on T2 imaging (Fig. 8.4).

The first follow-up evaluation at 3 months included MDCT imaging (Fig. 8.5), which depicted stable disease; however, over the same period there had been a significant decrease in the serum CA 19-9 level (from 567 to 146 IU/mL).

This case shows that DWI may have an important role in monitoring response to treatment. Rather than tumor shrinkage, the increased ADC can be considered indicative of cell death, as an early phenomenon that correlates better with the biochemical response (decrease in tumor markers) than with a size reduction at MDCT.

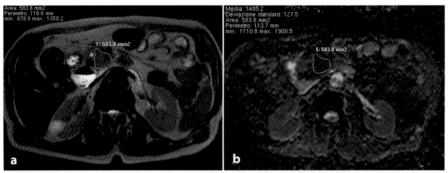

Fig. 8.3 a Pre-treatment T2-weighted MRI confirms the presence of a slightly hyperintense mass of the pancreatic head. **b** ADC map of the same region shows low signal intensity corresponding to the lesion. ADC value = $1.40 \pm 0.13 \times 10^{-3}$ mm^2/s

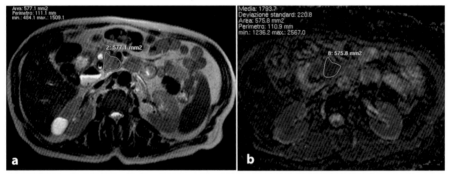

Fig. 8.4 After one month from the start of treatment, the lesion size is unchanged at MRI (**a**) but the ADC values are slightly increased (**b**). ADC value = $1.79 \pm 0.22 \times 10^{-3}$ mm^2/s

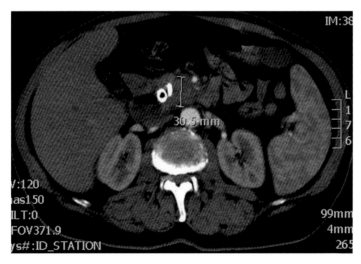

Fig. 8.5 No significant changes can be observed at MDCT, performed 3 months after the start of chemotherapy, compared to the pre-treatment scan

References

1. Sultana A, Tudur Smith C, Cunningham D et al (2007) Systematic review, including meta-analyses, on the management of locally advanced pancreatic cancer using radiation/combined modality therapy. Br J Cancer 96:1183-90
2. Cascinu S, Falconi M, Valentini V et al (2010) Pancreatic cancer: ESMO Clinical Practice Guidelines for diagnosis, treatment and follow-up. Ann Oncol 21:55–58
3. Reni M, Pasetto LM, Passardi A et al (2011) Treatment trends in metastatic pancreatic cancer patients: is it time to change? Dig Liv Dis 43:225-230
4. Reni M, Cordio S, Milandri C et al (2005) Gemcitabine versus cisplatin, epirubicin, 5-fluorouracil, gemcitabine in advanced pancreatic cancer: a phase III trial. Lancet Oncol 6:369-376
5. Reni M, Cereda S, Rognone A et al (2011) A randomized phase II trial of two different 4-drug combinations in advanced pancreatic adenocarcinoma: cisplatin, capecitabine, gemcitabine plus either epirubicin or docetaxel (PEXG or PDXG regimen) Cancer Chemother Pharmacol in press
6. Conroy T, Desseigne F, Ychou M et al (2011) FOLFIRINOX versus gemcitabine for metastatic pancreatic cancer. N Engl J Med 364:1817-1825
7. Kamisawa T, Isawa T, Koike M et al (1995) Hematogenous metastases of Pancreatic ductal carcinoma. Pancreas 11:345-349
8. Moertel CG, Childs DS jr, Reitemeier RJ et al (1969) Combined 5- fluorouracil and supervoltage radiation therapy of locally unresectable gastrointestinal cancer. Lancet 2:865-867
9. Moertel CG, Frytak S, Hahn RG et al (1981) Therapy of locally unresectable pancreatic carcinoma: a randomized comparison of high dose (6000 rads) radiation alone, moderate dose radiation (4000 rads+ 5-fluorouracil), and high dose radiation + 5-fluorouracil: The Gastrointestinal Tumor Study Group. Cancer 48:1705-1710
10. Klikenbijl JH, Jeekel J, Sahmoud T et al (1999) Adjuvant radiotherapy and 5- fluorouracil after curative resection of cancer of the pancreas and periampullary region: phase III trial of the EORTC gastrointestinal tract cancer cooperative group. Ann Surg 230:776-782, discussion: 782- 784
11. Neoptolemos JO, Dunn JA, Stocken DD et al (2001) Adjuvant chemoradiotherapy and chemotherapy in resectable pancreatic cancer: a randomized controlled trial. Lancet 358:1576-1585
12. Regine WF, Winter KA, Abrams RA et al (2008) Florouracil vs gemcitabine chemotherapy before and after florouracil- based chemoradiation following resection of pancreatic adenocarcinoma: a randomized controlled trial. JAMA 299:1019-1026
13. Brunner TB and Scott- Brown M (2010) The role of radiotherapy in multimodal treatment of pancreatic carcinoma. Radiation Oncology 5:64
14. Khanna A, Walker GR, Livingstone AS et al (2006) Is adjuvant 5-FU-based chemoradiotherapy for resectable pancreatic adenocarcinoma beneficial? A meta-analysis of an unanswered question. J gastrointestinal Surg 10:689-697
15. Stocken DD, Buchler MW, Dervensis C et al (2005) Meta-analysis of randomized adjuvant treatment therapy trials for pancreatic cancer. Br J Cancer 92:1372-1381
16. Gillen S, Schuster T, MeyerZum Buschenfelde C et al (2010) Preoperative/neoadjuvant therapy in pancreatic cancer: a systematic review and meta-analysis of response and resection percentages. Plos medicine 7(4):e1000267
17. Brunner TB, Grabenbauer GG, Meyer T et al (2007) Primary resection versus neoadjuvant chemoradiation followed by resection for locally resectable or potentially resectable pancreatic carcinoma without distant metastasis. A multi-centre prospectively randomized phase II-study of the Interdisciplinary Working Group Gastrointestinal Tumours (AIO, ARO and CAO). BMC Cancer 7:41

18. Chauffert B, Mornex F, Bonnetain F et al (2008) Phase III trial comparing intensive in-
     duction chemoradiotherapy (60 Gy, infusional 5-FU and intermittent cisplatin) followed
     by maintenenace gemcitabine with gemcitabione alone for locally advanced unresectable
     pancreatic cancer. Definitive results of the 2000-01 FFCD/SFRO study. Ann Oncol 19:1592-
     1599
19. Loehrer PJ, Powell ME, Cardenes HR et al (2008) A randomized phase III study of gemc-
     itabine in combination with radiation therapy versus gemcitabine alone in patients with lo-
     calized, unresectable pancreatic cancer: E4201. J Clin Oncol 26 (suppl:abstract 4506)
20. Haller DG (2003) New perspectives in the management of pancreas cancer. Semin Oncol 30:3-
     10
21. Huguet F, André T, Hammel P et al (2007) Impact of chemoradiotherapy after disease con-
     trol with chemotherapy in locally advanced pancreatic adenocarcinoma in GERCOR phase
     II and III studies. J Clin Oncol 25:326-331
22. Verweij J, Therasse P, Eisenhauer E, RECIST Working Group (2009) Cancer clinical trial out-
     comes: any progress in tumour-size assessment? Eur J Cancer 45:225-227
23. Rezai P, Mulcahy MF, Tochetto SM et al (2009) Morphological analysis of pancreatic ade-
     nocarcinoma on multidetector row computed tomography: implications for treatment re-
     sponse evaluation. Pancreas 38:799-803
24. Suzuki C, Jacobsson H, Hatschek T et al (2008) Radiologic measurements of tumor response
     to treatment: practical approaches and limitations. Radiographics 28:329-344
25. Reni M, Cereda S, Balzano G et al (2009) Carbohydrate antigen 19-9 change during chemother-
     apy for advanced pancreatic adenocarcinoma. Cancer 115:2630-2639
26. Hess V, Glimelius B, Grawe P et al (2008) CA 19-9 tumour-marker response to chemother-
     apy in patients with advanced pancreatic cancer enrolled in a randomised controlled trial. Lancet
     Oncol 9:132-138
27. Bünger S, Laubert T, Roblick UJ, Habermann JK (2011) Serum biomarkers for improved di-
     agnostic of pancreatic cancer: a current overview. J Cancer Res Clin Oncol 137:375-389
28. Choi M, Heilbrun LK, Venkatramanamoorthy R et al (2010) Using 18F-fluorodeoxyglucose
     positron emission tomography to monitor clinical outcomes in patients treated with neoadju-
     vant chemo-radiotherapy for locally advanced pancreatic cancer. Am J Clin Oncol 33:257-
     261
29. Park MS, Klotz E, Kim MJ et al (2009) Perfusion CT: noninvasive surrogate marker for strat-
     ification of pancreatic cancer response to concurrent chemo- and radiation therapy. Radiolo-
     gy 250:110-117
30. Akisik MF, Sandrasegaran K, Bu G et al (2010) Pancreatic cancer: utility of dynamic con-
     trast-enhanced MR imaging in assessment of antiangiogenic therapy. Radiology 256:441-449
31. Irie H, Honda H, Kuroiwa T et al (2002) Measurement of the apparent diffusion coefficient
     in intraductal mucin-producing tumor of the pancreas by diffusion-weighted echo-planar MR
     imaging. Abdom Imaging 27:82-87
32. Niwa T, Ueno M, Ohkawa S et al (2009) Advanced pancreatic cancer: the use of the appar-
     ent diffusion coefficient to predict response to chemotherapy. Br J Radiol 82:28-34
33. Orsi MA, Losio C, De Cobelli F et al (2009) Magnetic Resonance Imaging of Advanced Pan-
     creatic Adenocarcinoma: Monitoring the Response to Chemotherapy With Diffusion-Weight-
     ed Sequences. From the acts of the 33rd AISP Congress. J Pancreas (Online) 10(5 Suppl): 589-
     645

Hepatocellular Carcinoma

9

Franco Brunello and Andrea Veltri

9.1 Introduction

Hepatocellular carcinoma (HCC) is the third most common cause of cancer-related death among men and the sixth among women [1]. In Western countries, its incidence has invariably increased over the last several decades and it is expected to continue rising, although the etiological landscape, until now dominated by hepatotropic viruses, may change in favor of metabolic diseases that involve the liver [2]. HCC is, in fact, currently most often associated with liver cirrhosis and chronic infection/chronic hepatitis from viral B and C hepatitis but toxic/metabolic diseases (alcohol abuse, hemochromatosis, and non-alcoholic steatohepatitis associated with obesity and diabetes) seem to be closely linked to a higher risk of developing HCC [3-5].

Until the 1980s, the treatment of HCC was limited to surgical resection, although its feasibility and success were limited to a few patients with resectable tumor (because of late diagnosis) and a high rate of peri-operative mortality and morbidity (due to complications related to associated liver cirrhosis and a reduced ability to surgically manage these patients). Consequently, HCC was considered to be a disease invariably associated with a poor prognosis, and over a short time for the majority of patients. However, the situation has changed in the last 30 years, with the introduction of liver transplantation, refinements in liver resection techniques, and the appearance of new "mini-invasive" techniques for the local non-surgical ablation of HCC nodules, i.e., chemoembolization, alcohol injection, and radiofrequency.

Technical improvements in US equipment and in interventional devices together with the development of new medical skills (e.g., catheterization of

A. Veltri (✉)
Department of Radiology, Facoltà San Luigi Gonzaga, University of Turin,
Orbassano (Turin), Italy

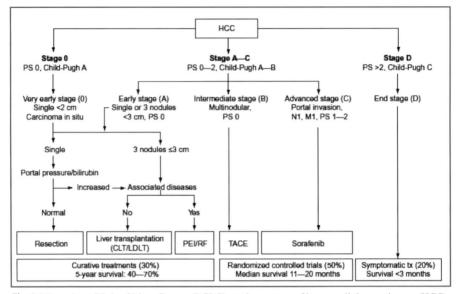

Fig. 9.1 Barcelona Clinic of Liver Cancer (BCLC) staging system of hepatocellular carcinoma (HCC). (Reproduced with permission from [8])

small hepatic arteries, ultrasound guidance of percutaneously introduced needles) have enlarged the possibilities for the safe treatment of patients previously not considered suitable for surgical resection or liver transplantation, thus modifying their prognosis. Moreover, early diagnosis has become more frequent following important technical improvements in the imaging tools themselves.

The choice of the "best" treatment must be tailored to each patient, depending upon individual features that may be associated in many different ways. Tumor burden, liver function, and performance status are the main clinical measures to be considered but also age, etiology of the underlying liver disease, previous diseases and surgical interventions, site of the lesion, lesion visibility, comorbidities and co-treatments.

In the Western world, the currently used staging system, endorsed by the European and American Societies for the Study of Liver Diseases (EASL and AASLD), is that of the BCLC (Barcelona Clinic of Liver Cancer). The BCLC system takes into account the three above-mentioned clinical features and classifies HCC into five stages: very early (0), early (A), intermediate (B), advanced (C), and terminal (D). For each stage, the algorithm suggests the "best" treatment as defined from evidence-based data available in the literature [6-9]. Figure 9.1 shows the general flow-chart of the BCLC staging system. It should be noted that the pathways indicated in the flow-chart are a simplification, and exceptions diverging from this scheme are frequently the "rule." Treatment for very early and early HCC will not be discussed.

Another noteworthy aspect is that, until a few years ago, the treatment of advanced HCC (stage C) lacked a definite and evidence-based approach. Previous empirically based treatments involving small non-randomized series of patients suggested mild benefit with combinations of various common chemotherapeutic agents such as tamoxifen, megestrol acetate, and octreotide. All these approaches have been successively abandoned; instead, sorafenib (discussed below), other newer target agents, and the more aggressive transarterial therapies are currently the best available options for patients with locally advanced disease. The following sections summarize the most relevant results as well as the limitations of these new therapies.

9.2   Transarterial Treatments

The embolization and chemoembolization of HCC nodules through their rich arterial feeding complex was proposed about 25 years ago, making it the first non-surgical treatment of liver cancer associated with cirrhosis [10, 11]. This percutaneous approach results in a brisk decrease in arterial feeding of the neoplasia, thereby inducing a more or less lasting ischemia and, in turn, severe damage and necrosis of the neoplastic tissue. Transarterial embolization (TAE) is performed by injecting into the right or left hepatic arteries (or, better, in a segmental hepatic artery where the tumor is located) various synthetic (Gelfoam, Ivalon, others) or natural (fibrin clots) particles that embolize the corresponding arterial tree. The same approach may be preceded by the intraarterial injection of an emulsion of lipoidol ultrafluid (LUF) oil vehiculating antineoplastic agents (doxorubicin, epidoxorubicin, cisplatin, 5-fluorouracil), with the latter ensuring additional chemotoxic damage to the tumor (transarterial chemoembolization, TACE). TACE has been recently modified to include the arterial injection of plastic or glass microspheres (300–500 μm in diameter) carrying themselves the chemotherapeutic agent. These charged beads embolize the small neoplastic arteries and then slowly release the toxic agent (DC-beads-TACE) [12, 13]. Neither intra-arterial chemotherapy (by pump), nor the intra-arterial injection of LUF + chemotherapeutic agents, nor lipiodolization alone achieve arterial occlusion and all three are therefore largely ineffective. For these reasons, today, they as well as other, traditional agents are rarely used for the treatment of HCC.

Alternatively, TAE and TACE have been proposed using different approaches (monolobar, simultaneous bilobar, segmental) and different strategies (scheduled treatments at 3–4 months or "on demand"). Some studies have noted the paradoxical decrease in the survival time of patients with non-optimal liver function who undergo TAE or TACE in a simultaneous bilobar approach [14]. Thus, nowadays selective/superselective segmental TACE is performed whenever possible in order to reduce the risk of toxic damage to the cirrhotic liver surrounding the neoplastic nodules. Nonetheless, clear evidence supporting a clinical benefit of TACE was lacking for many years after its introduction into clinical practice. Finally, however, two randomized controlled trials demonstrated the effectiveness, in terms of overall survival, of TACE (not of TAE) performed through the segmental approach in patients with multifocal disease but with good or relatively well preserved liver function [15, 16]. TACE has therefore become the standard treatment for patients suffering from liver cirrhosis and multifocal intermediate-stage HCC (BCLC class B, occasionally C) [17]. Both traditional and DC-beads-TACE yield a highly variable (16–60%) local response of the treated nodules [11, 17]. However of the two options, DC-beads-TACE has been demonstrated to induce less severe collateral effects (post-TACE syndrome) due to the slow release of chemotherapeutic agent [18].

A technical variation of TACE is radio-embolization (TARE). This technique, originally based on the injection of a radionuclide (^{131}I) LUF emulsion into the arterial hepatic system, initially yielded promising results in some patients but was then largely abandoned [19]. However, TARE has lately regained some of its interest because of the recent introduction of new embolizing agents, i.e., the above-described glass or plastic beads, linked to the β-emitting radionuclide ^{90}Y [20, 21]. With this new approach, radio-insulated rooms and radio-protected waste disposal systems are no longer necessary. Indeed, yttrium is not eliminated through the feces or the urine and its range of action is limited to a few millimeters around the nodule treated by radioactive embolization. Although a clear advantage compared to TACE in terms of overall survival has not yet been demonstrated, TARE may be useful in patients with advanced-stage disease in which there is also lobar neoplastic portal thrombosis (a contraindication for TACE), as thrombus regression with portal revascularization has been observed. In this setting, TARE may be considered a potential competitor of sorafenib; however, to date, it is not considered a standard treatment for HCC and its use should be limited to selected cases [22].

9.3   Targeted Therapies

Until a few years ago, there was no single chemotherapeutic agent or combinations of different agents (intravenously or intra-arterially injected) providing effective medical treatment of HCC in non-surgical patients [23]. Yet, with advances in the field of targeted therapies, there is support for the use of sorafenib, an oral multikinase inhibitor with anti-proliferative and anti-angiogenic effects in renal cell carcinoma, as an effective treatment for HCC as well [24, 25].

Sorafenib acts by blocking the Raf/MEK/ERK pathways, the receptor of vascular endothelial growth factor receptor (VEGFR 2), and the platelet-derived growth factor receptor β (PDGFR-β) [25]. Since HCC is a malignancy characterized by intensive arterial neovascularization, it is potentially responsive to the inhibition of related pathways and receptors [26]. A phase II study [27] demonstrated the clinical usefulness of the drug in patients with cirrhosis and HCC. Successively, the efficacy of sorafenib was examined in two large phase III randomized, double-blind, controlled trials (the SHARP Study [28] and the Asia-Pacific Study [29]), in different (Western and Eastern) populations, with respect to disease that differed in etiologic prevalence. In these patients with advanced-stage HCC and liver cirrhosis, the endpoints were the achievement of a median overall survival of 3 months and disease progression benefits. The most frequent adverse events were hand-foot syndrome reaction, diarrhea, and fatigue [28]. In patients who received the drug, median overall survival was 10.7 months, whereas in patients given the placebo overall survival was 7.9 months (HR 0.69; 95% CI 0.55–0.87; $p < 0.001$). The median time to progression was 5.5 months vs. 2.8 months (HR 0.58; 95% CI 0.45–0.74; $p < 0.001$). Based on these results, sorafenib has become the standard of care for patients suffering from advanced HCC (BCLC C). Two comprehensive clinical reviews dedicated, respectively, to sorafenib and targeted therapies of HCC were recently published [30, 31].

Several trials now in progress are aimed at determining whether other agents (epidermal growth factor, insulin-like growth factor, fibroblast growth factor, c-MET, mTOR inhibitors, and other VEGFR and Raf inhibitors) are able to induce a stronger antitumoral effect than sorafenib while maintaining a similar or better safety profile. Thus far, no other targeted therapy has achieved these results. Ongoing phase III (STORM) and phase II (SPACE) studies of patients with early- and intermediate-phase HCC treated with TACE or resection/ablation are expected to generate information about the clinical usefulness of sorafenib in earlier stages of HCC. Preliminary data from these studies should be available within the next 2 years.

Aside from its demonstrated beneficial effects on survival and time to progression, sorafenib may induce objective signs of tumor regression, mainly the devascularization of HCC nodules but also a reduction in tumor burden or the regression of neoplastic thrombosis. These results are seen in a minority of patients (2–4%) whereas stabilization of the tumor burden and slowed progression are the rule. No marker predictive of the response to sorafenib is available to date and patients have to be strictly followed by imaging techniques in order to recognize those who are not responders, allowing them to be withdrawn from a useless and expensive treatment. Sorafenib-resistant patients should instead be referred to those specialized centers where trials on new targeted treatments, either alone or in combination with sorafenib, are now the focus of phase II or phase III trials.

Thus, overall, the treatment of HCC involves agents and strategies with very different actions. In some cases tumor shrinkage demonstrates the activity of the treatment whereas with the new targeted therapies a delay in tumor progression and more subtle changes in tumor imaging most often comprise the main therapeutic results. Acknowledging this fact is of paramount importance: indeed, we are entering an era in which conventional radiological assessment may not always be adequate, reflecting the growing need to tailor the imaging technique to the type of treatment.

9.4   Imaging Response to Treatment in Locally Advanced HCC

9.4.1   Monitoring Response Using Conventional Radiological Assessment

As reported above, according to the BCLC staging system, locally advanced HCC might coincide with stages B (intermediate), C (advanced), or D (terminal). In the case of intermediate cancer, the current standard of care is chemoembolization (TACE) (Fig. 9.2), while targeted therapies are preferred in advanced cases [9]. Locoregional treatments are mostly intra-arterial, but percutaneous ablation can be performed in combination with TACE either to extend necrosis in the larger lesions or to treat smaller satellite lesions. Targeted therapies integrated with TACE are being evaluated in clinical studies, mostly in the context of preventing recurrence.

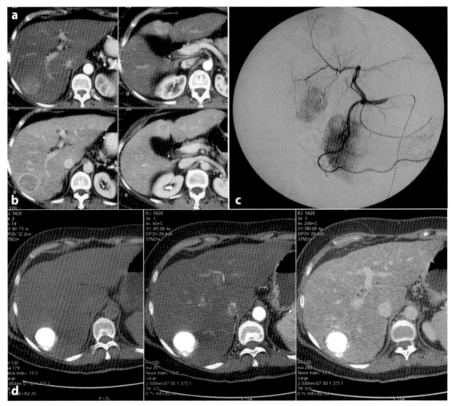

Fig. 9.2 Intermediate (BCLC) stage HCC (multinodular, at least one nodule > 3 cm in diameter). **a, b** Pre-treatment CT shows two liver nodules with arterial-phase enhancement and washout in the delayed phase. **c** Arteriography during chemoembolization (TACE) confirms CT findings. **d** Post-TACE triphasic CT scan (pre-contrast, arterial, and delayed phases) shows complete uptake of iodized oil by the HCC and the absence of intravenous contrast medium enhancement in the arterial phase, both signs of a good treatment result

In all these situations, apart from the timing, the follow-up imaging protocol is very similar to the one recommended by the EASL and AASLD for initial staging (Fig. 9.3).

According to the AASLD guidelines, suspicious liver nodules > 1 cm should be investigated either with multi-phase, multi-detector computed tomography (MDCT) or dynamic contrast-enhanced MRI (DCE-MRI). If the vascular profile is not typical of HCC (i.e., hypervascular in the arterial phase with washout in the portal venous or delayed phase; Fig. 9.2), a second contrast-enhanced study with the other imaging modality should be performed, or the lesion should be biopsied.

The same document contains a subchapter titled "Monitoring Response to Treatment," in which the authors state that the efficacy of treatment should be monitored radiologically. Successful treatment is defined as a lack of vascular enhancement within the lesion, and tumor recurrence in the treated area or elsewhere as the re-appearance of vascular enhancement. Thus, post-treatment monitoring should also be performed with contrast-enhanced imaging, either CT or MRI (Fig. 9.2), as to date there is no evidence that one modality is superior to the other.

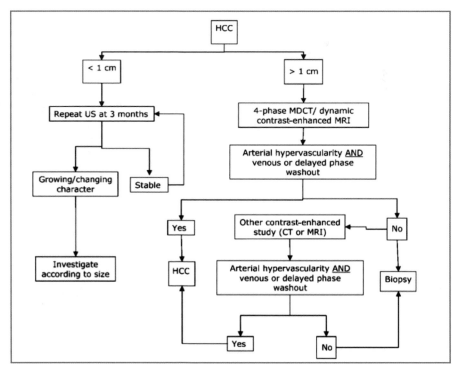

Fig. 9.3 Algorithm for the investigation of HCC nodules. (Reproduced with permission from Hepatology, Wiley-Blackwell, John Wiley & Sons, [9])

In 2008, the Italian National Guideline System produced a document on the diagnostic imaging of focal hepatic lesions (http://www.snlg-iss.it/cms/files/LG_Diagno_01-64_2008.pdf). It stated that CT and MRI are the techniques of choice at the 3-month follow-up of patients who have undergone oncological treatment. In particular, CT and MRI are recommended after radiofrequency thermal ablation and percutaneous ethanol injection, and MRI after TACE.

Two aspects of the above-mentioned guidelines should be highlighted. The first is that contrast-enhanced ultrasound (CEUS) is certainly cost-effective when evaluating the reduction of vascularization in hypervascular HCC hours and days after treatment; the second is that in the evaluation of residual enhancement, MRI is preferred over CT after TACE with LUF, due to the absence of interference with the oily contrast medium. Nevertheless, among the above-mentioned techniques, CT remains the most frequently used in the restaging and monitoring of all treated lesions.

In 2009, the Society of Interventional Radiology (SIR) also specified the role of imaging in monitoring the response to treatment in the field of Interventional Oncology. In the general paper on tumor ablation, which dealt with local, mostly thermal treatments, the role of imaging was discussed with respect to the assessment of treatment response immediately after completion of the procedure and during the follow-up period [32]. In the first scenario, the important recommendations noted the significance of the ablation zone. Indeed, the post-procedural imaging findings are defined as "only a rough guide" to the success of ablation therapy, since it is unlikely that microscopic foci of residual disease will be identified. Treatment may induce a series of imaging findings including those related to zones of decreased perfusion within the lesion and those related to peri-lesional findings (i.e., transient hyperechoic zone, benign peri-ablational enhancement, irregular peripheral enhancement, involution of coagulation, etc.). The SIR guidelines also specify the timing of imaging during follow-up. Contrast-enhanced CT or DCE-MRI should be performed within 6 weeks of the initial ablation, to determine whether additional ablation therapy is required, and thereafter every 3–4 months, to determine effectiveness. As noted by the authors, the correct evaluation of treatment results should not simply rely on size criteria but, at least, must also take into account the differences in tumor enhancement. In fact, according to the statement of the International Working Group on Image-Guided Tumor Ablation, "… given the heavy reliance on morphologic features other than size in the assessment of results of ablation therapy, exclusive reliance on tumor size does not provide a complete imaging assessment of tumor response and may even lead to erroneous conclusions about the effectiveness of the therapy. Therefore, in addition to reporting index tumor and the zone of ablation diameters, assessment of tumor enhancement or lack thereof should also be included in the imaging response assessment following ablation therapy."

In 2009, the SIR also published two papers on intra-arterial treatment. In the first, which focused on post-procedural imaging [33], the importance of CT and MRI signs in the evaluation of the treatment results was stressed, particularly the CT signs of tumor necrosis, including iodized oil uptake and the absence of arterial-phase enhancement in areas where it was present before chemoembolization (Fig. 9.2). In fact, the disappearance of arterial enhancement was defined as the principal determinant of tumor necrosis on MRI. However, the difficulty of evaluating the treatment of hypovascular HCC was noted. In such cases, size criteria must be relied upon, considering gross enlargement in the setting of residual or recurrent tumor after chemoembolization as a sign of progression. In the second paper [34], the two above-mentioned effectiveness criteria were reaffirmed: the uptake of iodized oil in HCC (a recommended scale is a five-grade system: no uptake, < 10% uptake, 10–50% uptake, > 50–99% uptake, complete uptake) and the absence of arterial-phase enhancement on cross-sectional imaging (Fig. 9.2). Initial evidence points to a favorable correlation between the increased uptake of iodized oil and survival. Nevertheless, due to the absence of significant validation studies, the authors of these papers finally stated that investigators should continue to rely on WHO or RECIST criteria. This assessment was explained in great detail, clarifying, above all, the differences between its significance in oncology and its applicability in monitoring HCC response to transcatheter therapy, thus indicating the need for modified RECIST criteria for HCC ("Complete radiologic response differs from the standard definition of complete response in trials of systemic therapies, which requires complete disappearance of the tumor... Residual disease may be represented by incomplete replacement of a HCC with iodized oil or persistent arterial-phase enhancement on CT or MR identified before and after treatment... Given that the response to transcatheter therapy can be non-uniform, change in diameter rather than contrast enhancement is considered to be the hallmark of progression... It is important to note that no or minimal regression does not imply treatment failure"). In conclusion, these recommendations point out both the difficulty in evaluating response to treatment in patients with locally advanced HCC and the substantial absence of standardized criteria until 2009.

9.4.2   Innovative Ways to Monitor HCC Response to Treatment: The mRECIST Assessment

As described in the previous section, the treatment of intermediate and advanced HCC is still largely experimental, due to the lack of strong evidence concerning the effectiveness of current therapies and to the development of innovative locoregional techniques and new drugs. Furthermore, it is now clear that imaging criteria, including the RECIST criteria, need to be adapted to the special features of HCC. Thus, in 2010, Lencioni and Llovet reported a set of guidelines developed by a group of experts convened by the AASLD, aimed at providing a common framework for the design of clinical trials [35]. These AASLD-JNCI (Journal of the National Cancer Institute) guidelines were the first to include a formal modification of the assessment of response based on

Table 9.1 Assessment of target lesion response following mRECIST amendments for HCC. Reproduced with permission from Semin Liver Dis, Thieme [35]

RECIST	mRECIST for HCC
CR = Disappearance of all target lesions	CR = Disappearance of any intratumoral arterial enhancement in all target lesions
PR = At least a 30% decrease in the sum of the diameters of target lesions, taking as reference the baseline sum of the dimeters of target lesions	PR = At least a 30% decrease in the sum of diameters of viable (enhancement in the arterial phase) target lesions. taking as reference the baseline sum of the diameters of target lesions (Fig. 9.4a)
SD = Any cases that do not qualify for either partial response or progressive disease	SD = Any cases that do not qualify for either partial response or progressive disease
PD = An increase of at least 20% in the sum of the diameters of target lesions, taking as reference the smallest sum of the diameters of target lesions recorded since treatment started	PD = An increase of at least 20% in the sum of the diameters of viable (enhancing) target lesions, taking as reference the smallest sum of the diameters of viable (enhancing) target lesions recorded since treatment started (Fig. 9.4b)

the RECIST criteria, and they sought to translate the concept of viable tumor, posed by the previous guidelines, in a more updated framework. These amendments were referred as the modified RECIST assessment (mRECIST) for HCC. Differences between RECIST amd mRECIST criteria are summarized in Table 9.1.

According to the new mRECIST criteria, patients can be followed with contrast-enhanced CT or dynamic MRI. In image interpretation, uniform image acquisition parameters and rigorous quality control are recommended. Baseline imaging should be performed to determine the overall initial tumor burden and used as the basis of comparison in subsequent measurements. Overall response assessment should include, similar to RECIST, an evaluation of target lesion response, non-target lesion response, and the presence of new lesions (see Table 2.1, Chapter 2). Target lesions should be selected on the basis of their size (those with the longest diameter) and their suitability for accurate repeated measurements. All other lesions (or disease sites) should be identified as non-target lesions and should also be recorded at baseline. Measurements of these lesions are not required, but the presence or absence of each one should be noted throughout follow-up. The measurement of the longest viable tumor diameter for the assessment of response according to mRECIST is to be applied only to typical lesions. Conversely, for non-enhancing atypical lesions, the measurements of the longest overall tumor diameter as per conventional RECIST should prevail. According to the panel of experts, a target lesion is to be selected using mRECIST, with an HCC lesion not only meeting the RECIST criteria (i.e., to be accurately measurable in at least one dimension as 1 cm or more and suitable for repeat measure-

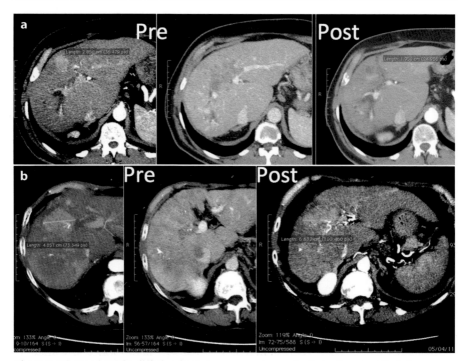

Fig. 9.4 Advanced HCCs differing in their response to sorafenib treatment. **a** Partial response after sorafenib treatment. Pre-treatment staging CT scans shows a target lesion (well-delineated, hypervascular in the arterial phase) and invasion of both the right and left portal branches. At restaging, the target lesion showed a 30% decrease in viable tissue (enhancing in the arterial phase) compared to the baseline. **b** Post-sorafenib progressive disease. A target lesion with a diameter of 4.8 cm was identified at the pre-treatment arterial-phase CT study. In the venous phase, portal and inferior vena cava invasion are observed due to direct infiltration by the HCC. A 20% increase of the diameter of the viable target lesion occurred during follow-up

ment), but also showing intratumoral arterial enhancement on contrast-enhanced CT or MRI. Moreover, only well-delineated, arterially enhancing lesions can be selected as target lesions for mRECIST. This may not be the case of infiltrative-type HCC, which should be considered as a non-target lesion when the mass shows ill-defined borders.

Similar to the RECIST assessment, in mRECIST the evolution of non-target lesions and the appearance of new lesions must be taken into account ("The appearance of one or more new lesions and/or unequivocal progression of existing nontarget lesions should declare progressive disease"). For the special features of HCC in cirrhosis, in the evaluation of non-target lesions particular attention must be paid to portal thrombosis, adenopathies of the hepatic hilum, and the appearance of pleural effusion and ascites. Furthermore, the characterization of a newly detected focal liver nodule as true HCC follows the

Table 9.2 Overall assessment in mRECIST for HCC. Reproduced with permission from Semin Liver Dis, Thieme Medical [35]

Target Lesions	Nontarget Lesions	New Lesions	Overall Response
CR	CR	No	CR
CR	IR/SD	No	PR
PR	Non-PD	No	PR
SD	Non-PD	No	SD
SD	Any	Yes or no	PD
Any	PD	Yes or no	PD
Any	Any	Yes	PD

mRECIST, modified Response Evaluation Criteria in Solid Tumors; *CR*, complete response; *PR*, partial response; *IR*, incomplete response; *SD*, stable disease; *PD*, progressive disease.

same diagnostic criteria as the already mentioned AASLD practice guidelines for the clinical management of HCC [9]. Lastly, the authors specified the mRECIST overall patient response criteria as a result of the combined assessment of target lesions, non-target lesions, and new lesions (Table 9.2).

It is too early to know whether the new mRECIST criteria provide a reliable method for assessing the response to treatment of intermediate and advanced HCC. Indeed, mRECIST based on the AASLD-JNCI guidelines could align the response rates induced by molecular drugs (namely, novel drugs currently tested in phase II and phase III studies) to hard endpoints, such as patient survival. However, against this background of ongoing discussions on the use of these new criteria of response to treatment, a new field of research is opening up, one that mainly deals with innovative radiological techniques. Among these, CT perfusion and diffusion-weighted imaging (DWI) are currently considered the most promising in evaluating treatment response, with respect to TACE and to anti-angiogenic therapies [36-39]. Responding HCC lesions exhibit changes in ADC values at DWI that sometimes are unusual [40]. CEUS has also been investigated in evaluating the response to new targeted-therapies, but more limited results are thus far available [39]. CT perfusion and CEUS reveal early changes in tumor perfusion that may be predictive of tumor response. Finally, ^{18}F-FDG PET is not considered in the algorithm for diagnosing and staging HCC [9], because the overall sensitivity of this modality in the detection of HCC is too low. Indeed in well-differentiated HCC, FDG metabolism may be similar to that of the surrounding liver, leading to a false-negative result, while higher sensitivity is reported for poorly differentiated HCC. Nonetheless, some authors have recently suggested the use of PET/CT to assess the early response to sorafenib in advanced HCC and as a biomarker with predictive and prognostic value in patients with positive scans at baseline [41, 42].

Clinical Case

In May 2009, a 61-year-old physically active male patient suffering from liver cirrhosis was evaluated for a 3-cm liver nodule in segment 6, detected at ultra-sonography. A quadriphasic CT scan of the upper abdomen confirmed a liver tumor of 3 cm in segment 6; the imaging features of the lesion were typical for HCC (hyperdensity in arterial phase with washout and hypodensity in late phases). The α-fetoprotein level was 50 ng/ml.

The patient was an HCV carrier who had never been treated. He was also positive for antibodies to HBcAg and HBsAg. His intake of alcoholic beverages was null. An upper endoscopy was not performed because he showed no signs of portal hypertension (splenomegaly, low platelet count, enlargement of spleno-portal veins). His liver function was excellent (Child-Pugh A/5).

His past history was uneventful except for two urologic interventions (small vesical papilloma and urolithiasis), mild arterial hypertension, and atopic dermatitis with eosinophilia.

The man refused surgical intervention, the best choice for this case of "early HCC," and was soon after treated by a single session of radiofrequency ablation (July 2009).

One month later, at CT follow-up performed to evaluate the results of treatment, a complete response of the treated lesion was determined (Fig. 9.5) and no new liver lesions were detected. However, a 27-mm pulmonary lesion was incidentally detected in the subpleural space of the dorsal segment of the right

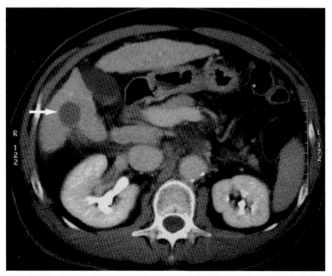

Fig. 9.5 In August 2009 portal phase axial CT scan show no vital tissue at the site of the HCC treated with radiofrequency ablation (*white arrow*)

inferior lobe. PET/CT confirmed the lung lesion and the patient underwent CT-guided fine-needle biopsy. Histology revealed adenocarcinoma and the patient underwent right pulmonary lobectomy. The final diagnosis was bronchioalveolar adenocarcinoma of the lung without nodal metastases.

In December 2009, a second CT of the upper abdomen confirmed the complete response of the lesion treated by radiofrequency, with two small doubtful lesions in the right lobe of the liver. In February 2010, an MRI study of the liver showed four small lesions (12–13 mm) typical for HCC in segments 6, 7, 8, and 2. The patient's disease was restaged as "intermediate HCC" and treated by conventional chemoembolization (TACE) of the right lobe. During the arteriographic phase, four lesions were in fact detected but all were located in the right lobe. No lesions were observed in segment 2 at angiography.

A CT scan performed 2 months later showed no active lesions in the right lobe, confirming the optimal results of TACE. However, a 45-mm hyperarterialized infiltrative lesion was clearly visible in segment 2; a neoplastic thrombus of the portal peduncle of segment 2 was also evident (Fig. 9.6).

In August 2010, the patient, now with "advanced HCC," started treatment with sorafenib (800 mg/day). The drug was well tolerated and after 1 month an ultrasound scan showed a partial dimensional regression of the active lesion in segment 2. Beginning in November 2010, the sorafenib was maintained at a reduced dosage (400–600 mg/day) because of recurrent diarrhea.

The CT scans performed in October 2010, January 2011, and May 2011 showed devascularization and progressive reduction, until complete disappearance, of the lesion in segment 2 and of the portal neoplastic thrombus (Fig. 9.7).

As of August 2011, one year from the beginning of sorafenib treatment, the patient is alive, in good clinical condition, and without any CT-detectable active lesion. There has been no recurrence of the concomitant lung tumor.

This clinical cases summarizes the fast evolution of HCC, which in 2 years went from being an early-stage surgical candidate to intermediate and finally advanced disease. Luckily, at all stages the patient responded optimally to treatment. The disease was probably multifocal in origin and surgical resection would have been followed by early recurrence. Liver transplantation was not a good indication initially because of the HCV etiology of his liver cirrhosis and a few months later it became contraindicated due to the occurrence of the pulmonary adenocarcinoma.

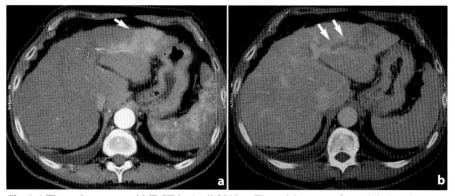

Fig. 9.6 The patient repeated MDCT in April 2010. **a** The axial scan performed during the arterial phase shows a 45 mm infiltrative hypervascular lesion of segment 2 (*white arrow*). **b** In the venous phase a neoplastic thrombus of the portal peduncle of segment 2 was also evident (*white arrows*)

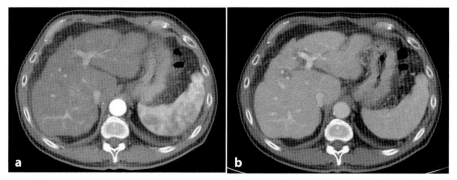

Fig. 9.7 The CT scans performed following therapy with sorafenib shows good response to treatment. **a** The axial CT in the arterial phase shows no enhancement; **b** in the portal phase the lesion is smaller and a regression of the portal vein thrombus is observed

References

1. Ferlay J, Shin HR, Bray F et al (2010) Estimates of worldwide burden of cancer. GLOBO-CAN 2008. Int J Cancer 127:2893-917
2. Nordenstedt H, White DL, El-Serag HB (2010) The changing pattern of epidemiology in hepatocellular carcinoma. Dig Liver Dis Suppl 3:S206-14
3. Bugianesi E, Leone N, Vanni E et al (2002) Expanding the natural history of nonalcoholic steatohepatitis: from cryptogenic cirrhosis to hepatocellular carcinoma. Gastroenterology 123:134-140
4. Starley BQ, Calcagno CJ, Harrison SA (2010) Nonalcoholic Fatty Liver Disease and Hepatocellular Carcinoma: A Weight Connection. Hepatology 51:1820-1832
5. Stroffolini T, Trevisani F, Pinzello G et al (2011) Changing pattern of hepatocellular carcinoma in Italy and implication for surveillance. In press on Digestive and Liver Dis
6. Bruix J, Sherman M, Llovet JM et al (2001) Clinical management of hepatocellular carcinoma. Conclusions of the Barcelona-2000 EASL Conference. J Hepatol 35:421-430
7. Bruix J, Sherman M (2005) Management of hepatocellular carcinoma. Hepatology 42:1208-1236
8. Llovet JM, Di Bisceglie AM, Bruix J et al (2008) Design and end points of clinical trials in hepatocellular carcinoma. J Natl Cancer Inst 100:698-711
9. Bruix J, Sherman M (2011) Management of hepatocellular carcinoma. An update. Hepatology 53:1020-2
10. Yang CF, Ho YJ (1992) Transcatheter arterial chemoembolization for hepatocellular carcinoma. Cancer Chemother Pharmacol 31 (Suppl):S86-8
11. Bruix J, Sala M, Llovet JM (2004) Chemoembolization for hepatocellular carcinoma. Gastroenterology 127 (Suppl):S179-188
12. Varela M, Real MI, Burrel M et al (2007) Chemoembolization of hepatocellular carcinoma with drug eluting beads: efficacy and doxorubicin pharmacokinetics. J Hepatol 46:474-481
13. Poon RT, Tso WK, Pang RW et al (2007) A phase I/II trial of chemoembolization for hepatocellular carcinoma using a novel intra-arterial drug-eluting bead. Clin Gastroenterol Hepatol 5:1100-1108
14. Group d'Etude e de Traitment du Carcinome Hepatocellulaire (1995). A comparison of lipiodol chemoembolization and conservative treatment for unresectable hepatocellular carcinoma. N Engl J Med 332:1256-1261
15. Lo CM, Ngan H, Tso WK et al (2002) Randomized controlled trial of transarterial lipiodol chemoembolization for unresectable hapatocellular carcinoma. Hepatology 35:1164-1171
16. Llovet JM, Real MI, Montaña X et al (2002) Arterial embolisation or chemoembolisation versus symptomatic treatment in unresectable hepatocellular carcinoma: a randomized controlled trial. Lancet 359:1734-1739
17. Llovet JM, Bruix J(2003) Systematic review of randomized trials for unresectable hapatocellular carcinoma: chemoembolization improves survival. Hepatology 37:429-442
18. Lammer J, Malagari K, Vogl T et al (2010) Prospective randomized study of doxorubicin-eluting bead embolization in the treatment of hepatocellular carcinoma: results of PRECISION V study. Cardiovasc Intervent Radiol 33:41-52
19. Raoul JL, Boucher E, Roland V et al (2009) 131-iodine Lipiodol therapy in hepatocellular carcinoma. Q J Nucl Med Mol Imaging 53:348-55
20. Salem R, Lewandowski RJ, Atassi B et al (2005) Treatment of unresectable hepatocellular carcinoma with use of 90Y microspheres (TheraSphere): safety, tumor response and survival. J Vasc Inter Radiol 16:1627-1639
21. Sangro B, Bilbao JI, Boan J et al (2006) Radioembolization using 90Y-resin microspheres for patients with adavanced hepatocellular carcinoma. Int Radiat Oncol Biol Phys 66:792-800
22. Forner A, Ayuso C, Real MI et al (2009) Diagnosis and treatment of hepatocellular carcinoma. Med Clin 132:272-286
23. Lopez PM, Villanueva A, Llovet JM (2006) Systematic review: evidence-based management

of hepatocellular carcinoma - an updated analysis of randomized controlled trials. Aliment Pharmacol Ther 23:1535-1547

24. Wilhelm S, Carter C, Lynch M et al (2006) Discovery and development of sorafenib: a multikinase inhibitor for treating cancer. Nat Rev Drug Discov 5:835-844

25. Wilhelm SM, Carter C, Tang L et al (2004) BAY 43-9006 Exhibits broad spectrum oral antitumor activity and targets the RAF/MEK/ERK pathway and receptor tyrosine kinases involved in tumor progression and angiogenesis. Cancer Res 64:7099-109

26. Schoenleber SJ, Kurtz DM, Talwalkar JA et al (2009) Prognostic role of vascular endothelial growth factor in hepatocellular carcinoma: systematic review and meta-analysis. Br J Cancer 100:1385-1392

27. Abou-Alfa GK, Schwartz L, Ricci S et al (2006) Phase II Study of Sorafenib in patients with advanced hepatocellular carcinoma. J Clin Oncol 24:4293-4300

28. Llovet JM, Ricci S, Mazzaferro V et al (2008) Sorafenib in advanced hepatocellular carcinoma. N Engl J Med 359:378-390

29. Cheng AL, Kang YK, Chen Z et al (2009) Efficacy and safety of sorafenib in patients in the Asia-Pacific region with advanced hepatocellular carcinoma: a phase II randomized, double-blind, placebo-controlled trial. Lancet Oncol 10:25-34

30. Finn RS (2010) Drug Therapy: Sorafenib. Hepatology 51:1843-1869

31. Villanueva A, Llovet JM (2011) Targeted therapies for hepatocellular carcinoma. Gastroenterology 140:1410-1426

32. Goldberg SN, Grassi CJ, Cardella JF et al (2009) Image-guided Tumor Ablation: Standardization of Terminology and Reporting Criteria. JVIR, 20(S), S377–S390. SIR. doi:10.1016/j.jvir.2009.04.011

33. Brown DB, Cardella JF, Sacks D et al (2009) Quality improvement guidelines for transhepatic arterial chemoembolization, embolization, and chemotherapeutic infusion for hepatic malignancy. JVIR, 20(S), S219–S226.e10. SIR. doi:10.1016/j.jvir.2009.04.033

34. Brown DB, Gould JE, Gervais DA et al (2009) Transcatheter Therapy for hepatic malignancy: standardization of terminology and reporting criteria. JVIR, 20(S), S425–S434. SIR. doi:10.1016/j.jvir.2009.04.021

35. Lencioni R, Llovet JM (2010). Modified RECIST (mRECIST) Assessment for Hepatocellular Carcinoma. Seminars in Liver Disease 30:52–60. doi:10.1055/s-0030-1247132

36. Ippolito D, Bonaffini PA, Ratti L et al (2010) Hepatocellular carcinoma treated with transarterial chemoembolization: dynamic perfusion-CT in the assessment of residual tumor. World J Gastroenterol, 16(47):5993-6000. doi: 10.3748/wjg.v16.i47.5993

37. Jiang T, Kambadakone A, Kulkarni NM et al (2012) Monitoring response to antiangiogenic treatment and predicting outcomes in advanced hepatocellular carcinoma using image biomarkers, CT perfusion, tumor density, and tumor size (RECIST). Invest Radiol 47:11-17. doi: 10.1097/RLI.0b013e3182199bb5

38. Sahin H, Harman M, Cinar C et al (2012) Evaluation of treatment response of chemoembolization in hepatocellular carcinoma with diffusion-weighted imaging on 3.0-T MR imaging. J Vasc Interv Radiol 23:241-247. doi:10.1016/j.jvir.2011.08.030

39. Schraml C, Schwenzer NF, Martirosian P et al (2009) Diffusion-weighted MRI of advanced hepatocellular carcinoma during sorafenib treatment: initial results. AJR 193:W301–W307. doi:10.2214/AJR.08.2289

40. Lassau N, Koscielny S, Chami L et al (2011) Advanced hepatocellular carcinoma: early evaluation of response to bevacizumab therapy at dynamic contrast-enhanced US with quantification-preliminary results. Radiology 258:291-300. doi:10.1148/radiol.10091870/-/DC1

41. Siemerink EJM, Mulder NH, Brouwers AH et al (2008) 18F-Fluorodeoxyglucose positron emission tomography for monitoring response to sorafenib treatment in patients with hepatocellular carcinoma. The Oncologist 13:734-735. doi: 10.1634/theoncologist.2008-0063

42. Lee JH, Park JY, Kim do Y et al (2011) Prognostic Value of 18F-FDG PET for hepatocellular carcinoma patients treated with sorafenib. Liver Int 31:1144-1149. doi: 10.1111/j.1478-3231.2011.02541.x

Printed in May 2012